Successful Breastfeeding

This handbook is dedicated with respect and affection to Dr Mavis Gunther. The members of the group have had to re-learn much of what Dr Gunther already knew in the 1940s, '50s and '60s; at last, in the 1980s, we were able to write the first edition of this handbook of breastfeeding which has been inspired by her sound clinical understanding and her rigorous scientific approach. We hope that we have continued in this tradition for the third edition.

For Churchill Livingstone:

Publishing Manager, Health Professions: Inta Ozols
Project Development Manager: Katrina Mather
Project Manager: Gail Murray
Designer: George Ajayi
Illustrators: Joanne Moon, Hilary English, Sylvia Barker, Mike Woolridge

Successful Breastfeeding

Third edition

Royal College
of Midwives

London 2002

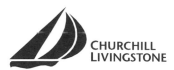

EDINBURGH LONDON NEW YORK PHILADELPHIA ST LOUIS SYDNEY TORONTO 2002

CHURCHILL LIVINGSTONE
An imprint of Harcourt Publishers Limited

Royal College of Midwives
15 Mansfield Street, London W1M 0BE

First edition 1988
Second edition 1991
Third edition 2002

ISBN 0 443 05967 5

British Library Cataloguing in Publication Data
A catalogue record for this book is available from the British Library

Library of Congress Cataloging in Publication Data
A catalog record for this book is available from the Library of Congress

Note
Medical knowledge is constantly changing. As new information becomes available, changes in treatment, procedures, equipment and the use of drugs become necessary. The authors and the publishers have, as far as it is possible, taken care to ensure that the information given in this text is accurate and up to date. However, readers are strongly advised to confirm that the information, especially with regard to drug usage, complies with the latest legislation and standards of practice.

The
Publisher's
policy is to use
**paper manufactured
from sustainable forests**

Printed in China

Contents

Preface   xii
Introduction   xiii
The background   xvii

1 Why breastfeed?   1
The limitations of breastmilk substitutes   1
Composition   2
Oils   3
Breast milk and substitutes compared   3
   Royal College of Midwives comparison chart   3
   Protein   4
   Free amino acids   6
   Cholesterol   6
   Fatty acids   6
   Carbohydrate   8
   Minerals   9
   Trace elements   9
   Bioavailability   10
Biologically different   10
Further issues   10
   Errors during manufacture   10
   Errors during preparation   11
   Controlling intake   12
   Nutritional summary   12
   Immunological factors   12
   Other substances   14
Disadvantages of bottle-feeding   14
   Health risks for the child   14
   Disadvantages for the mother   15
   Fertility   15
The economics of not breastfeeding   16

2 Understanding how a baby breastfeeds   23
Milk production and the role of lactational hormones   23
Colostrum and milk production in the first week of life   24
   Colostrum   24
   Milk volume   25
   Milk removal   25
Feedback inhibition of lactation   27
Milk release and infant 'sucking'   27
Changes in the breast during pregnancy and parturition   33
Variations in breast size   33

Contents

3 Duration and frequency of feeds 36

Duration of feeds 36
Frequency of feeds 37
   Initiation of breastfeeding 37
   Range of feed frequencies from the first week onwards 37
Variability in intake/infant appetite 39

4 Correct positioning and attachment of the baby at the breast 41

Introduction 41
The different appearances of breast- and bottle-feeding 41
When to offer help to the mother 43
Steps to achieving correct attachment 43
Indications that the baby is properly attached 49
Ways in which the midwife can help directly 51
Postural considerations 53
   Suggestions for the first feed 53
   Helping the mother to feed lying down 53
   Helping the mother to feed sitting up 56
   Position and posture of the midwife 57

5 Factors that have been shown to help 60

Advice and support at the first feed 60
Unrestricted feeds 63
   Unrestricted duration of feeds 63
   Unrestricted frequency of feeds 64
Feeding the baby at night 66
   The value of night feeds 66
   Rooming in 67
   Bedding-in 67
   The mother's sleep 69
Monitoring the baby's health and well-being 69
   Weight 70
   Weight gain 70
   Weight variations 71
   Stools 72
   General health 73

6 Factors that have been shown to be unhelpful 78

Additional fluids for breastfed babies 78
   Dehydration 78
   Jaundice 79
   Hypoglycaemia 79
   Hazards of additional fluids 80

Test weighing 81
Unsubstantiated 'advice' to mothers in relation to food,
drink and rest 82
    Additional fluids for breastfeeding mothers 82
    Additional calories for breastfeeding mothers 83
    Dietary prohibitions for breastfeeding mothers 84

7 Protecting breastfeeding **89**
Provision of free samples to mothers 89
Promotion of breastmilk substitutes 90
    WHO code 90
    Baby Friendly Hospital initiative and the Ten Steps 92

8 Antenatal and postnatal considerations **93**
Influencing the decision to breastfeed 93
    Antenatal classes 94
Sustaining the decision to breastfeed 95
Prevention of feeding problems 96
    Antenatal preparation 96
    Nipple shape 97
    Nipple preparation 97
Postnatal care of the breasts 98
    Cleanliness 98
    Creams and ointments 98
    Limiting sucking time 99
Treatment of sore nipples 99
    Resting, expressing and repositioning (reattachment) 100
    Damaged nipples and moist wound healing 101
    Nipple shields 101
Hand expression 102
    How to help a mother to hand express 102
Prevention and treatment of engorgement 103
    Vascular engorgement 103
    Milk engorgement 104
    Prevention of engorgement 104
    Treatment 104
Prevention and treatment of mastitis 105
    Non-infective mastitis 106
    Infective mastitis 106
    Prevention of non-infective mastitis 106
    Prevention of infective mastitis 107
    Treatment of mastitis 107

9 Notes on less common problems 115

Baby vomiting blood or digested blood in stools 115
Blood in milk or colostrum 115
Blanching of the nipple (white nipple) 116
Thrush infection 116
Contact dermatitis 117
Diabetes 117
Epilepsy 117
Anticoagulant therapy 117
Other drugs and breastfeeding 117
Mammary surgery 118
Cleft lip 118
Cleft palate 118
Down syndrome 119
Tandem feeding 119
Breast abscess 119
Inverted nipples 119
HIV and breastfeeding 120
Hepatitis B 121
Hepatitis C 121
Herpes simplex infection 121

10 Breastfeeding under special circumstances 124

Preterm infants 124
HIV and milk banking 125
Caesarean section 126
Twins 126
Triplets 127
Establishing lactation with an electric pump 127
How to help a mother express using an electric pump 128
Silicone inserts for pump collection kits 129
Storage of breast milk or colostrum 129
Alternatives to bottle-feeding 130
Babies being cared for in units other than maternity units 131

Appendix 1: The Ten Steps to Successful Breastfeeding 134

Appendix 2: National and international voluntary organisations 135

Appendix 3: Breastfeeding initiatives in the UK 138

Appendix 4:   Further reading   144

Appendix 5:   Health benefits of breastfeeding   146

Appendix 6:   Royal College of Midwives
comparison chart   152

Index   151

Preface

A breastfeeding working group was set up by the Council of the Royal College of Midwives in May 1986, in response to a challenge issued by the December 1985 meeting of the Royal Society of Medicine's Forum on Maternity and the Newborn. The subject of that meeting was 'Difficulties with Breastfeeding – Midwives in Disarray?' (Inch 1987). There it was acknowledged that for a variety of reasons there was very little consistency between breastfeeding policies in different parts of the country and also between policy and practice within many individual institutions. Furthermore, it was apparent that many current practices (and policies) were not only unsupported by research evidence but in some cases contradicted by it. It was the hope expressed there that midwives, the main professional body concerned with breastfeeding, would take the lead in establishing a working party (which would include broad representation from other bodies) in order to ascertain what the current evidence suggested was good practice, to which members of the RCM Council have responded.

At that time, the principal members of the working group were Chloe Fisher (Senior Midwife, Oxford), Sally Garforth (Midwife, Reading), Sally Inch (Midwife, Oxford, who has acted as chief editor for this edition of *Successful Breastfeeding*), Ellena Salariya (Research Midwife, Dundee) and Michael Woolridge (Research Fellow, Department of Child Health, Bristol). Jean Rowe (Health Visitor, London) and Margaret Kerr (Midwife, Northern Ireland) also contributed to the final document.

The group gratefully acknowledges the help and advice received from Evelyn Elliott (National Childbirth Trust), Rachel O'Leary (La Leche League) and Peggy Thomas (Association of Breastfeeding Mothers), who attended most of the working group's meetings, and Phillipa Cardale (RCM Serving Officer for the group), who tactfully and efficiently administered the group.

Thanks are due to all those who read and commented on the various drafts of the first edition of the handbook, and to the new contributors to the third edition, Hilary English and Dora Henschel.

The second edition was available worldwide and so far has been translated into: Catalan, Castilian, German, Swedish, Norwegian, Danish, French and Bosnian.

Reference
Inch S. Difficulties with breastfeeding – midwives in disarray? Report of the 11th Meeting of the Royal Society of Medicine's Forum on Maternity and the Newborn 1987. Journal of the Royal Society of Medicine 1987; 80:53–58.

Introduction

This handbook has been written to help midwives, and others, provide more effective advice and support for the breastfeeding women in their care.

Human milk has evolved over many thousands of years to meet the specific needs of human infants, just as the milk of all other mammals has evolved to meet the specific needs of their young. Not surprisingly, therefore, the more that is known about the nutritional, immunological and other properties of breast milk, the more superior it appears in comparison with all other available milks for human babies.

The introduction to the first two editions of *Successful Breastfeeding* 'regarded it as axiomatic that...all babies should be exclusively breastfed until they are at least four, and preferably six months old'. In keeping with the current climate of 'informed choice' and 'evidence-based practice' this edition contains a new section that lists the specific benefits of breastfeeding to both mothers and babies. Midwives need to be presented (as does every other group of health professionals) with the fullest discussion of the differences between breast milk and commercially available substitutes, so that they can make an informed choice. Health professionals who are unaware of these differences will not be able to help women make a fully informed choice, and may not have the motivation to acquire the skills needed to enable women who choose to breastfeed to do so successfully.

The majority of women in Great Britain (68%) now choose to breastfeed (Foster et al 1997). In spite of this only a minority (28%) are still fully breastfeeding at 4 months, which is the minimum duration recommended at the time these data were compiled (Department of Health 1994).

Many women abandon breastfeeding during the first 2 weeks (Foster et al 1995) when the mother and her baby are still in the care of midwives. The World Health Organization has accepted that the vast majority of women (97% or more) are physiologically capable of breastfeeding their babies successfully (Chetley 1986). The discrepancy between those who are capable and those who succeed may pinpoint weaknesses among those who support them rather than the women themselves. Indeed, one Australian writer attributes a large part of the responsibility for breastfeeding failure to professional ignorance (Minchin 1998). She continues (pp. 44–45):

'I am not imputing negligence or stupidity or malice, or making any other moral judgements. I know that most professionals are hard working, humane and dedicated. I am reporting that there is a degree of professional ignorance which is historically quite understandable, but no longer tolerable.'

Teaching a mother breastfeeding skills may lack the glamour and urgency of intrapartum care, but it is an integral part of a midwife's role and can be equally rewarding. Furthermore the midwife, as the key health worker in the early postnatal days, has the opportunity and privilege of making a tremendous difference to the experience and success of breastfeeding women.

However, every woman who has started to breastfeed her baby, and every midwife who has tried to help, will be familiar with the widespread experience of conflicting advice (Beeken & Waterston 1992), to which the Report of the Maternity Services Advisory Committee (Maternity Care in Action 1985) drew attention, and which was reinforced in *Changing Childbirth* (Department of Health 1993). It is hoped that this handbook will overcome the conflict in the advice given to breastfeeding women, as it bases its recommendations for practice on sound research evidence.

The need to achieve consistency and rationality in the support given by midwives and other staff is even more important in view of the difficulties imposed by the present system of care. Ideally, a mother and her baby would receive all their care from one skilled individual. However, most women still have their babies in a hospital where there is a shift system of staff for postnatal care.

This is compounded by the present economic restraints within the health service which often result in a midwife being responsible for as many as 30 mothers and babies at a time in hospital, and in selective visiting being practised in the community. Consequently the time available to help each individual woman establish breastfeeding is severely restricted. It is therefore crucial that the advice and support that midwives can offer is the best available and that it is constantly reinforced by all their colleagues.

The needs of the baby have been adequately met, in most cases, by the intricate physiological mechanisms of the mother's body during the months spent in utero. The mother's breasts can provide a fluid that is equally intricate, and precisely tailored to her baby's extrauterine needs. No other food can match it, and the possible short- and long-term consequences of depriving babies of breast milk are only just beginning to be investigated.

In recognition of the importance of breastfeeding to both mothers and babies, this handbook is offered as both a resource and a practical guide for midwives. It begins with a brief outline of the history of breastfeeding in Britain since the beginning of the twentieth century, and thus an explanation for the fact that so many midwives found themselves ill equipped to assist breastfeeding women. The remainder of the handbook is consequently devoted to providing sound, research-based information to increase their knowledge, skill and confidence.

The first section deals with the differences, in both composition and effect, between breast milk and breastmilk substitutes on the health and well-being of the infant.

The second section explains the physiology of breastfeeding, as a thorough understanding of this is vital for providing effective care. This is followed by a detailed description of how to attach a baby to the breast correctly, as this basic midwifery skill is fundamental to breastfeeding success.

Many of the issues in breastfeeding practice, such as the regulation of feeds or the use of supplementary fluids, are then examined in the light of current research findings. Practices that have been shown to help women breastfeed are recommended, and those that may hinder success are identified.

Finally it is recognised that problems and special circumstances do occur. Where appropriate, the origins of common problems are discussed, along with effective prevention and treatment.

Notes

1. We acknowledge that babies are either male or female but, as all mothers are female, we have, for the sake of clarity, referred to the baby as he or him throughout.
2. Unless otherwise stated, it should be assumed that the baby is a healthy term infant.
3. Throughout the text 'positioning' will refer to the relationship of the baby's body to the mother's body, and 'attachment' to the relationship of the baby's mouth to the breast.

References

Beeken S, Waterston A. Health service support of breastfeeding – are we practising what we preach? BMJ 1992; 305:285–287.

Chetley A. The politics of babyfood – successful challenges to an international marketing strategy. London: Francis Pinter; 1986 (in which Chetley quotes the World Health Organisation's provisional summary record of the 8th meeting of Committee A, 33rd World Health Assembly; document no. A33/A SR/8; Geneva, 17 May 1980, p. 11).

Department of Health. Changing childbirth. Report of the Expert Maternity Group. London: HMSO; 1993.

Department of Health. Weaning and the weaning diet. Report on Health and Social Subjects, 45. London: HMSO; 1994.

Foster K, Lader D, Cheesbrough S. Infant feeding 1995. London: The Stationery Office; 1997.

Maternity Care in Action. Report of the Maternity Services Advisory Committee Part 3. Care of mother and baby (postnatal and neonatal care). 1985; p. 5.

Minchin M. Breastfeeding matters. What we need to know about infant feeding. Melbourne: Alma Publications, 1998.

The background

At the beginning of the twentieth century there was growing concern about the future of the 'British Race'. The high infant mortality rate, 153 per 1000 live births (Newman 1931), was causing great concern and was thought to be the result of two major factors: artificial feeding (Howarth 1905) and the 'ignorance and fecklessness of mothers' (Lewis 1980).

The medical profession's response to this was to try to make artificial feeding 'scientific' and therefore safer. There followed a short but intense period of interest in the composition and preparation of bottle-feeds; and a small number of doctors emerged as 'experts' on infant feeding, about which they wrote prolifically. Unfortunately their books also contained much advice about breastfeeding, a subject on which it was assumed, erroneously, that they would be equally knowledgeable.

Two ideas originated at this time, neither of which appears to have been seriously questioned subsequently. The first was that the breastfed baby fed from the nipple, as if it were similar to a teat on a bottle, rather than from the breast. Breastfeeding was thus thought to be traumatic to the nipple and mothers were strongly advised to restrict the duration of feeds in the first few days in order to prevent nipple damage (King 1913). It was also believed that as there was 'only a small amount of colostrum' it would take the baby a short time to consume it, and that 'sucking on an empty breast' would also make the nipple sore (*Midwifery by Ten Teachers*; Berkeley 1920). The sixteenth edition of this same textbook, *Obstetrics by Ten Teachers*, published in 1995, still recommends short initial feeds (Chamberlain 1995).

The second idea, which probably originated in Europe (Budin 1907), was that severe 'digestive disorders' were likely to be the result of 'overfeeding' breastfed babies. The medical 'experts' thus invented rules relating to the frequency with which a baby should be fed, in order to try to prevent this condition. These 'new' breastfeeding rules appeared in textbooks so repetitively that they soon became widely accepted practices, the reader undoubtedly assuming that they were scientifically based.

These ideas were also disseminated in the 'schools' that were set up for the 'ignorant' mothers. More importantly, they also started to appear in midwifery textbooks. *Mayes' Handbook of Midwifery* is an excellent example, for in the first edition, published in 1937, a rigid schedule for both the early feeds and subsequent feeds was recommended. This continued throughout the following nine editions over a period of nearly 44 years, with only slight variations. It is also interesting to note other recommendations in the handbook during this period. 'Until breastfeeding is established, which may take up to four weeks, complementary or even supplementary feeds may be necessary' (Thomas 1953, p. 283). 'For the first two or three nights an artificial feed is given by the midwife. This allows the mother to have a good rest. After this she may, if she wishes, give the child a breastfeed when he wakes' (Bailey 1967, p. 326). How outdated these ideas appear at the beginning of the twenty-first century.

As early as 1938, two British doctors were already protesting at this 'modern' management. Waller (1938, pp. 139–140) wrote:

'The harm done nowadays is not confined to turning out badly trained nurses but extends to the mothers who easily are led to believe that feeding is less an affair of technique than a sum in arithmetic, and that if their babies don't thrive at the breast when "clocked in" and "clocked out" like factory hands, the sooner they are fed artificially and by measure the better. Neither realises that it is this absurd guidance by the clock which already constitutes artificial feeding; artificial because, applied without understanding, it takes no account of the physiology of lactation or of the emotional side of motherhood, and overlooks the baby's dependence on both if it is to thrive.'

The second author (Spence 1938, pp. 730–731) wrote:

'The essence of the faults in most hospitals and nursing homes is that they attempt too much to mechanise breast-feeding. They have institutional rules about times of feeding, the amount of the feeds, the weighing of babies, and the test weighing of feeds, to which they try to fit the patient.'

At this time most women were giving birth at home and they continued to breastfeed as they had always done, with their friends and relatives supporting, advising and handing down the art of breastfeeding. Women who were better off, however, gave birth in nursing homes and hospitals under the care of doctors, and were thus taught the new rules. Coincidentally, medical writers began to comment on the inability of upper-class women to breastfeed successfully, a fact which they attributed to the effects of 'higher civilisation' (Vincent 1904). Within a few years of their origin, the rigid rules had become firmly established in most hospitals, despite the misgivings of the Ministry of Health (1943), and more and more women were exposed to them as hospital births increased. (By the 1960s, when breastfeeding levels reached an all-time low, most women were giving birth in hospital.)

A measure that revealed the concern felt about the importance of breastfeeding early in the twentieth century was a new regulation that was included in the Central Midwives Board (CMB) rules of 1919 requiring notification by midwives of any case of cessation of breastfeeding during the statutory lying-in period (Lewis 1980). This requirement was withdrawn from the rules of the CMB in 1960. A comment in the *Midwives Chronicle and Nursing Notes* reporting this change stated: 'This seems a sensible change in view of modern ideas on infant feeding' (1960). It is not surprising that an editorial in the journal *Maternal and Child Care* (Mullins 1968, p. 220) under the heading 'Is breastfeeding finished?' should end with this paragraph:

'A paediatrician we know has for years campaigned to persuade mothers to breastfeed. To encourage them he has a fine collection of artistic reproductions, both old and new, showing every conceivable variety of breastfeeding. Now that the battle is virtually over and lost, he has the comfort and joy of his beautiful and interesting collection which might one day, we feel, form the basis of a recorded history of a past biological phenomenon.'

Dried cow's milk, which was produced for the government during the Second World War as an alternative and readily available method of infant feeding, continued to be supplied cheaply – or even free – by the newly formed welfare state, as National Dried Milk; this may also have contributed to the decreased incidence of breastfeeding. As fewer and fewer mothers breastfed, both mothers and midwives lost their skills in the art of breastfeeding.

Because of changes in both society and the place of birth, many families do not now have continuous and consistent support from relatives and neighbours. For this reason many women are more dependent on midwives and breastfeeding counsellors for support than ever before. It is thus of the utmost importance, for the sake both of the women in their care and of the profession, that midwives strive to improve their knowledge of, and skills in, breastfeeding. Supporting women in initiating and establishing breastfeeding is the one part of the midwife's role to which no other health professional can lay claim.

References
Bailey R, ed. Mayes' handbook of midwifery. 7th edn. London: Baillière Tindall; 1967 (also 8th edn, 1972; 9th edn,1976).

Berkeley Sir C. Midwifery by ten teachers. 2nd edn. London: Edward Arnold; 1920.

Budin P. The nursling. London: Caxton; 1907.

Chamberlain G, ed. Obstetrics by ten teachers. 16th edn. London: Edward Arnold; 1995.

Howarth WJ. The influence of feeding on mortality of infants. Lancet 1905; ii:210–213.

King FT. Feeding and care of the baby. New Zealand: Society for the Health of Women and Children; 1913.

Lewis J. The politics of motherhood. London: Croom Helm; 1980.

Mayes' handbook of midwifery. London: Baillière, Tindall & Cassell; 1937.

Midwives Chronicle and Nursing Notes Sept 1960; LXXIII (837):310

Ministry of Health. Reports on Public Health and Medical Subjects no 91. Report on the breast feeding of infants. London: HMSO; 1943.

Mullins A, ed. Is breastfeeding finished? Maternal and child care, vol IV London: Bouverie Publishing; Nov 1968.

Newman G. Health and social evolution. London: George Allen & Unwin; 1931.

Spence JC. The modern decline of breast-feeding. BMJ 1938; 2(4057): 729–733.

Thomas FD, ed. Mayes' handbook of midwifery. 4th edn. London: Baillière, Tindall & Cox; 1953 (also 5th edn, 1955; 6th edn, 1957).

Vincent R. The nutrition of the infant. London: Baillière, Tindall & Cox; 1904.

Waller H. Clinical studies in lactation. London: William Heinemann; 1938.

Why breastfeed?

The limitations of breastmilk substitutes	1
Composition	2
Oils	3
Breast milk and substitutes compared	3
Biologically different	10
Further issues	10
Disadvantages of bottle-feeding	14
The economics of not breastfeeding	16

'When comparisons are being made with breastmilk, an appeal of "no contest" should be recognised. Natural selection is an optimising process, and the controlled trial for breastmilk, with human survivability as the outcome measure, has been in progress for a minimum of 240,000 years – or 8000 generations' (Woolridge 1991)

Human milk is a species-specific fluid of great complexity, which has evolved over time to optimise the growth and development of the young for a vast array of short- and long-term outcomes. Breastmilk substitutes, on the other hand, which have been available commercially for a mere 150 years or so, aim to provide adequate nutrition and to maximise growth, with the consequence that children fed these substitutes are heavier at the end of the first year of life than their breastfed counterparts (Dewey et al 1992). Bottle-fed babies are also much less likely to be, or to have been, in good health (Inch 2000, UNICEF, WHO, UNESCO 1989).

The limitations of breastmilk substitutes

Although they may have come a long way since the mid-nineteenth century and Liebig's 'perfect infant food' – which was made from wheat flour, cow's milk, malt flour, pea flour and bicarbonate of potash (Palmer 1988) – the fact remains, and will always remain, that 'breastmilk substitutes' can only ever imitate the substances in breast milk if they are identifiable, if the technology exists to synthesise them, and if it is economic to synthesise them.

Composition

Although minimum and maximum permitted levels of named ingredients for artificial milks for infants are laid down by statute (Infant Breastmilk Substitutes and follow-on regulations 1995, statutory instrument 1995 no. 77), precisely what goes into breast-milk substitutes is increasingly being questioned by researchers.

Recommendations for the upper and lower limits of nutrients are often based on limited data, data from adults or data from other species (Walker 1993). Until 1984 recommendations for the amounts of calcium, phosphorus and magnesium were too high because they were based on information derived in 1953. Other important nutrients currently added were absent; either because they were not thought necessary, such as zinc and cysteine, or because they had yet to be identified. It was not until 1984 that taurine, now known to be essential for the myelination of the central nervous system, was added to all breastmilk substitutes (Minchin 1985). Before that, infants fed taurine-free milk had to use other amino acids as substitutes in the formation of their cerebellum, visual cortex and retina.

Changes are constantly being made to breastmilk substitutes – at least 100 every year (Messenger 1994). All infants consuming the breastmilk substitutes prior to the change or addition received food deficient in the substances newly defined as being essential for optimal growth and development.

In any case, adding new ingredients has to be done with caution. As the base product to which they are added is extensively processed, unexpected interactions can occur, resulting in further problems. For example, adding vitamin D to prevent rickets (partly caused by the poor absorption of calcium from earlier breastmilk substitutes) resulted in hypercalcaemia (Arnold et al 1985, Stapleton et al 1957).

Large amounts of iron are still added to breastmilk substitutes: about 20 times the concentration found in breast milk. This is because in the absence of the iron-binding protein, human lactoferrin, iron is not well absorbed by infants. Furthermore the percentage of iron absorbed decreases in inverse proportion to the amount added (i.e. the more iron added, the smaller the proportion absorbed) (Dallman 1989). At the same time, these larger amounts may inhibit the absorption of zinc and copper, and favour the development of pathogenic gut bacteria, some of which, ironically, may cause sufficient gut damage and microscopic bleeding to produce iron deficiency anaemia (Oski 1985).

Oils

Commercial considerations are also bound to influence the composition of breastmilk substitutes. For example, when the price of corn oil rose, soya and coconut oils were mixed with it (Food and Chemical News 1980). If it made economic sense, whale oil or pig fat could equally well be used, provided the fatty acid composition was satisfactory (Brooke 1985). Currently the only oils specifically prohibited by the 1995 Regulations are sesame seed or cotton seed oil, or fats containing more than 8% *trans*-isomers of fatty acids.

Breast milk and substitutes compared

Comparisons of the composition of breast milk and some of the common Western breastmilk substitutes are widely available, many of them from the manufacturers. What is not apparent from the usual listing of constituents by category is the structural and qualitative differences between them.

Royal College of Midwives comparison chart
The only comparison chart that begins to highlight the differences, rather than the similarities, between breast milk and the commonly used substitutes was published by the RCM in 1994.

Table 1.1

Per 100 mL	Breast	Gold	Premium	Firstmilk	Aptamil
Energy (kcal)	70	65	66	68	67
Protein (g)	0.9	1.5	1.4	1.45	1.5
Fat (g)	4.2	3.6	3.6	3.82	3.6
Carbohydrate (g)	7.3	7.2	7.5	7.0	7.3

Sections of this chart are reproduced in Tables 1.1–1.4 and the full chart can be found in Appendix 6.

Protein

Mature human milk has a lower protein concentration than that of any other mammal (Akre 1989) and provides an appropriately low solute load for the immature kidney. The higher protein intake provided by breastmilk substitutes results in raised blood urea and amino acid levels, and thus higher renal solute levels. (Raiha et al 1986). Neither the short- nor the long-term consequences of this increased metabolic stress are yet known. The higher protein concentration available in breastmilk substitutes offers no advantage in terms of growth and places the infant at a higher risk of hypernatraemic dehydration in situations that reduce body water, such as hot weather, fever or diarrhoea (Walker 1993).

The human whey proteins consist mainly of human α-lactalbumin, which is an important component of the enzyme lactose synthetase. The dominant bovine whey protein, on the other hand, bovine β-lactoglobulin, has no human-milk protein counterpart and is capable of provoking antigenic responses in atopic infants. The incidence of such allergy in the first year of life ranges from 2% to 7.5% of artificially fed infants (Adler & Warner 1991, Bahna 1987).

Another bovine whey protein, bovine serum albumin, has been implicated as the trigger for the development of insulin-

Table 1.2

Per 100 mL	Breast	Gold	Premium	Firstmilk	Aptamil
α-Lactalbumin	✔✔✔✔	(bovine)	(bovine)	(bovine)	(bovine)
β-Lactoglobulin	✘	✔✔✔	✔✔✔	✔✔✔	✔✔✔
Lactoferrin	✔✔	Trace	Trace	Trace	Trace
Immunoglobulins (mainly IgA)	✔✔	Trace	Trace	Trace	Trace
Lysozyme	✔✔	Trace	Trace	Trace	Trace
Casein (micelle structure)	Soft curds	Hard curds	Hard curds	Hard curds	Hard curds

dependent diabetes mellitus (IDDM) (Karjalainen et al 1992, Monte et al 1994); this may explain the fact that infants fed breastmilk substitutes have a 1.5–2-fold increased risk of developing IDDM than breastfed infants (Virtanen et al 1991).

The other main whey proteins present in human milk, lactoferrin, immunoglobulins and lysozyme, play important roles in protecting the infant from disease. In the presence of immunoglobulin (Ig) A antibody and bicarbonate, human lactoferrin (not present in bovine milk) can absorb enteric iron, thus depriving potentially pathogenic organisms (such as *Escherichia coli*, *Salmonella* and *Candida albicans*) of the iron they need to survive (Riordan 1993).

A large number of other proteins present in low concentrations in human milk (enzymes, growth modulators and hormones) are also absent from breastmilk substitutes.

The concentration of casein, another of the protein components of milk, varies widely between different mammals. Its molecular structure is characterised by the formation of micelles containing calcium and phosphorus, which makes it a good source of these minerals (Hambraeus 1977).

When exposed to pH changes or certain enzymes, casein forms curds. Human milk with its low (predominantly β) casein content forms small, soft, flocculent curds which are digested easily by the infant, thus supplying a continuous flow of nutrients.

Table 1.3

Per 100 mL	Breast	Gold	Premium	Firstmilk	Aptamil
Cystine: methionine ratio	1.3:1	0.7:1	0.6:1	0.6:1	0.6:1
Cholesterol (important in infancy)	16 mg	✗	✗	✗	✗
Linoleic: linolenic ratio	9.1:1	10.5:1	5.1:1	7.3:1	10.8:1
DHA* & AA**	✔✔	✗	✗	✗	✔✔

* DHA, docosahexaenoic acid. ** AA, arachadonic acid;

Breastmilk substitutes based on cow's milk, with their higher (and predominantly α) casein content, form larger, firm curds which stay in the infant's stomach for longer and require a higher expenditure of energy for complete digestion (Daniels 1989, Riordan 1993, Worthington-Roberts 1993). If the reconstituted powder is inadequately diluted, this curd complex of insoluble calcium caseinate, calcium phosphate and fat may be so dense as to cause intestinal obstruction (Jelliffe & Jelliffe 1978, Wales et al 1989).

Free amino acids

Human milk has higher levels of cystine, and lower levels of methionine, than does cow's milk. The cystine:methionine ratio of human milk is unique for animal tissues and one-seventh of that found in cow's milk (Jelliffe & Jelliffe 1978). This has implications for optimal brain development, particularly in the preterm infant in whom the necessary enzyme (cystothionase) required to convert methionine to cystine may be absent. High levels of methionine may adversely affect the central nervous system (Worthington-Roberts 1993).

Cholesterol

Cholesterol is present in human milk at much higher levels than in cow's milk or commercial infant breastmilk substitutes. It appears to play a part in the myelin synthesis of the rapidly growing nervous system. It has also been suggested that its presence in breast milk stimulates the development of enzymes necessary in later life for cholesterol degradation (Jelliffe 1975, Joote et al 1991).

Fatty acids

As well as cholesterol, human milk also contains small amounts of phospholipids, mono- and di-glycerides, glycolipids, other sterol esters and free fatty acids, but 98% of the lipid in human milk is in the form of triglycerides, that is, three fatty acids linked (esterified) to a single molecule of glycerol (Hernell 1990). More than 100 individual fatty acids have been identified in human milk.

The fatty acid composition of human milk is relatively stable, consisting of about 46% saturated and 54% unsaturated fatty acids (Jensen 1989).

In human milk many of these unsaturated fatty acids take the form of long-chain polyunsaturated fatty acids (LC-PUFAs), which are particularly important for brain growth and myelination. Two of the polyunsaturated fatty acids from which these longer-chain fatty acids are derived are linoleic and linolenic acid. These cannot be synthesised by the infant, nor the mother, who obtains them from dietary plant sources (Sinclair 1992).

However, the conversion from the parent fatty acid to the usable long-chain derivative, which in the case of linoleic acid includes arachadonic acid (AA) and in the case of linolenic acid includes docosahexaenoic acid (DHA), takes place rather slowly (Sinclair 1992). This is compensated for in the breastfed infant by the presence in human milk of the derivatives as well as the precursors

The infant who is not fed human milk, particularly if born prematurely, may not be able to convert the precursors to their biologically active form as fast as is needed for the developing brain and retinal membranes. In such circumstances other derivatives from the parent fatty acids may be used as substitutes, leading to markedly different concentrations of LC-PUFAs in the brain and retinal tissue (Farquharson et al 1992).

The debate begun in the early 1990s, which considered the value of adding LC-PUFAs to breastmilk substitutes, is still continuing. Although it is clear that, by comparison with breastfed babies, those fed artificially (particularly if preterm) are at a measurable disadvantage, the question is whether simply adding these fats to breastmilk substitutes will make any measurable difference (Crawford 1993, Lucas at al 1999, Makrides et al 1995). (It is also debatable whether mothers would be happy to feed their babies with derivatives from microalgae, fungi or tuna fish eye sockets (Martyn 1997).)

The ratio of linoleic to linolenic acid supplied in the milk may also create difficulties for artificially fed infants as an excessive intake of linoleic acid may itself inhibit α-linolenic metabolism (Farquharson et al 1992) because they compete for the same enzyme system (Hernell 1990).

The absorption of fats from the milk is facilitated by taurine, which conjugates bile acids. Infants who do not receive adequate amounts of taurine in their diet conjugate bile acids with glycine, which is less effective (Riordan 1993).

Fat digestion is also aided by the presence of a non-specific lipase, which is activated by bile salts in the infant's duodenum (Watkins 1985). Because it has no positional specificity, bile salt-stimulated lipase (BSSL) will hydrolyse all three ester bonds in triglycerides, and contribute to the digestion of mono-, di- and tri-glycerides as well as esterified fat-soluble vitamins (Hernell 1990). This is one more reason why net fat absorption is more efficient in preterm infants fed on breast milk than in those fed breastmilk substitutes.

This provision of both the substrate and its enzyme in the same fluid is a feature of human milk that is shared with only one other mammal – the gorilla (Akre 1989).

Carbohydrate

The carbohydrate component of human milk is provided chiefly by lactose, although small amounts of galactose, fructose and other oligosaccharides are also present.

Lactose is a sugar found only in milk and appears to be a nutrient specific to infancy: the enzyme lactase is found only in the young of all mammals except humans, in whom it may persist into adult life, particularly amongst Europeans. However, many of the world's people do not tolerate lactose after middle childhood (Akre 1989).

As well as providing about 40% of the energy needs of the infant, lactose facilitates calcium and iron absorption and encourages *Lactobacillus bifidus* to colonise the gut. This colon-

Table 1.4

Per 100 mL	Breast	Gold	Premium	Firstmilk	Aptamil
Calcium: phosphorus ratio	2.3:1	1.5:1	2.0:1	1.2:1	1.7:1
Zinc: copper ratio	7.6:1	10.0:1	8.1:1	8.4:1	8.7:1
Iron bioavailability (%)	70	10	10	10	10
Vitamins A B C D E K	Present	Added	Added	Added	Added

isation is further encouraged by the presence in human milk of a nitrogen-containing carbohydrate, the bifidus factor, which is absent from bovine milk derivatives.

In consequence, the pH in the gut is kept low (i.e. acid), and this discourages the replication of enteropathogens such as *Shigella*, *Salmonella* and some *E. coli*. The gut of infants fed breastmilk substitutes, which are subsequently colonised mainly with coliform and putrefactive bacteria, have a higher pH.

Minerals
Mineral concentrations are lower in human milk than in any breastmilk substitute. Whilst meeting the infant's nutritional needs because of their high bioavailability, minerals in breast milk also match the infant's metabolic capabilities.

Calcium is more efficiently absorbed from human milk than from breastmilk substitutes because of human milk's high calcium:phosphorus ratio. The high phosphorus content of breastmilk substitutes using bovine milk proteins has been reported to increase the risk of neonatal hypocalcaemic tetany in the first 10 days of life by a factor of 30 (to 30 in 10,000 from 1 in 10,000), possibly because the parathyroid gland is too immature to cope with it (Specker et al 1991).

Zinc, which is essential to enzyme structure and function, growth and cellular immunity, is present in human milk in small amounts which are sufficient to meet the needs of the infant without disturbing copper or iron absorption (Akre 1989) and is important in preventing infantile eczema.

Trace elements
Copper, along with other trace elements, cobalt and selenium, are, on the other hand, present at higher levels than in cow's milk.

The high bioavailability of copper in human milk, bound to proteins of low relative molecular mass, ensures that the breast-fed infant's needs are met. Copper deficiency occurs only in artificially fed infants (Akre 1989).

The ratio of copper to zinc in breastmilk is lower than that found in most breastmilk substitutes. High zinc:copper ratios have been associated with coronary heart disease in adults (Akre 1989).

Bioavailability

The higher bioavailability of minerals from human milk is the result of a complex series of interactions between the form in which the minerals are presented in the milk and the infant's body. In the case of iron, for example, appropriate levels of zinc and copper, the transfer factor, lactoferrin, and the higher acidity of the gastrointestinal tract combine to unlock the lactoferrin molecule, allowing up to 70% of the available iron to be absorbed. The iron in breastmilk substitutes is in the form of an inorganic salt, usually ferric ammonium citrate, only 10% of which is absorbed (Akre 1989, Williams 1993).

Biologically different

Ebrahim (1979, pp. 59–60) powerfully presented the fundamental nature of the differences between breastfeeding and the use of breastmilk substitutes in the following personal view:

'Infants who are fed artificially are biologically different from those who are breastfed. Their blood carries a different pattern of amino acids, some of which may be at levels high enough to cause anxiety. The composition of their body fat is different. They are fed a variety of carbohydrates to which no other mammalian species is exposed in neonatal life.

'They have higher plasma osmolarity, urea and electrolyte levels. Their guts are colonised by a potentially invasive type of micro flora, at the same time as they are exposed to large amounts of foreign protein resulting in an immunologic response. (In addition they are deprived of the immune factors present in human milk.) All these factors need to be taken into account every time a decision is made not to breastfeed an infant, for inherent in that decision are known and unknown risks to the infant.'

Further issues

Errors during manufacture

Infants fed breastmilk substitutes are disadvantaged not only by virtue of the intended constituents of the breastmilk substitutes, but also by factors associated with their production. All breastmilk substitutes have the potential for inadvertent excesses or deficiencies during the manufacturing process. There is also the danger of accidental contamination. Documented cases include contamination with aluminium, iodine, halogenated hydrocarbons and bacteria (Minchin 1985, Walker 1993).

As with any other manufactured food item, the possibility of deliberate contamination also exists.

Milk powder has also become contaminated as a result of interaction between the can and its contents, particularly with regard to lead and plasticisers (Minchin 1985, Walker 1980, Walker 1993).

Errors during preparation

The potential for error does not end with the manufacture of the breastmilk substitutes. Those who buy a substitute may use it inappropriately. This is most apparent where the purchaser cannot read the instructions on the tin or packet, either because they are illiterate or the instructions are in the wrong language. It may also be the case where parents have no reliable access to fuel, clean water or the means of sterilisation.

The cost of the breastmilk substitute may sometimes result in it being overdiluted to make it go further. At the other extreme, the use of microwave ovens in the preparation of feeds has resulted in the explosion of glass bottles (Signman-Grant et al 1992), burns to the mouth and throat of babies (Hibbard & Blevins 1988) and, under laboratory conditions, biochemical changes to the amino acids, producing toxic compounds that can damage the kidney, liver and brain (Lubec et al 1989).

In the more affluent West, feeds are often made up with too much powder for a given amount of water. Sometimes this is deliberate, when an extra scoop is added, supposedly to 'satisfy' the baby, but more commonly it is a result of inaccuracies in either the measuring scoop or the fact that the instructions either to level it off or not to pack it down differ from brand to brand.

The problem of accidentally over-concentrating feeds, which can result in obesity, intestinal obstruction, hyperna-traemia and other metabolic stresses, might be overcome if manufacturers supplied *only* packets containing a standard amount of dry powder, or bottles/cartons of ready-to-feed mixture, but that is likely to increase both the packaging and the price (Jeffs 1989, Lucas et al 1991, 1992).

Controlling intake

Finally, breastfed infants can control their calorie intake and their total food intake in a way that infants fed breastmilk substitutes cannot. The burst–pause sucking pattern of a breastfed infant differs from that of a bottle-fed infant, and their intake volume is relatively stable between 1 and 4 months of age, whereas infants fed breastmilk substitutes increase their intake volume over the same period (Montandon 1986). The first observation may be explained by the fact that an artificial feed is homogeneous, whereas the fat content of breast milk rises as the feed progresses; and the second by the fact that mothers control bottle-feeding, whereas babies control breastfeeding.

Nutritional summary

'To summarise...the situation with regard to...the nutrient content of breastmilk substitutes: we don't know exactly what ought to be in them; we can't guarantee that what we intend to put in will be exactly what we do put in; we don't know how to put it there in such a way that it will still be there when prepared for the child; nor can we guarantee that it will be made up by the user exactly as it should be...' (Minchin 1985, p. 11)

All that, however, is just the beginning, because breast milk is much more than a fluid providing optimal nutrition.

Immunological factors

The undisputed ability of human milk to protect the infant from a wide variety of pathogens – viral, parasitic and bacterial – is due to the presence of several groups of protective factors. Breast milk contains white cells (macrophages and lymphocytes), anti-inflammatory components, non-antibody factors, such as lactoferrin, the bifidus factor, enzymes such as lactoperoxidase and oligosaccharides, all of which also have other functions.

In addition, five types of immunoglobulin have been identified in breast milk: A, D, E, G and M, of which IgA predominates.

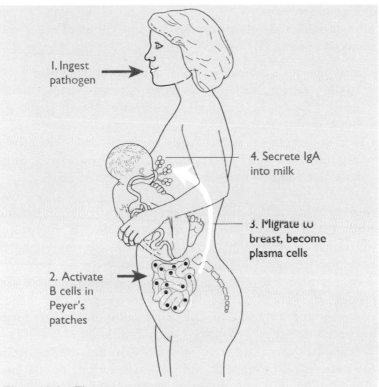

Figure 1.1 The entero-mammary system.

The mother's body is also able to monitor and respond to potential pathogens in her infant's environment from moment to moment via an elegant system known as GALT and BALT (gut-associated and bronchus-associated lymphoid tissue) or the broncho-mammary and entero-mammary circulation (Fig. 1.1).

Pathogens that enter the mother's respiratory or gastrointestinal tract stimulate pre-committed lymphocytes in the bronchial submucosa or in the Peyer patches of the small intestine. The activated β cells migrate via the blood to the mammary (and salivary) glands, where they become transformed into plasma cells which start secreting large quantities of the appropriate neutralising antibody into the milk (Newman 1995, Riordan 1993, Short 1994, Slade & Schwartz 1987, Worthington-Roberts 1993).

Other substances
Human milk and colostrum also contain a host of other substances including (Weaver 1997):

- enzymes, such as amylase, BSSL and lipoprotein lipase
- trophic factors, such as epidermal growth factor, human
  growth factors I, II and III, insulin-like growth factor and
  nerve growth factor
- anti-inflammatory agents and cytokines, such as prosta-
  glandin E and F, α1-antitrypsin, α1-antichymotrypsin, inter-
  leukins 1 and 6, interferon and tumour necrosis factor.

Also present are a variety of hormones including thyroxine,
adrenal and ovarian steroids, calcitonin, thyroid stimulating
hormone, thyrotrophin releasing hormone, adrenocorti-
cotrophic hormone, insulin, somatostatin, oxytocin, prolactin,
erythropoietin and prostaglandins. The presence of these hormones may account for the observed differences in the infant's
endogenous hormonal response to human milk compared with
breastmilk substitutes (Aynsley-Green 1983).

Some of the many enzymes so far identified are important
for neonatal development and cell maturation; others aug-
ment the infant's own digestive system, and still others are
bacteriolytic.

Disadvantages of bottle-feeding

Health risks for the child
Even in Western industrialised societies, some children pay the
ultimate price for being bottle-fed. The US National Institute of
Environmental Health Sciences estimated in 1989 that four of
every 1000 babies born in the USA will die each year because
they are not breastfed (Rogan 1989). In the UK, Lucas & Cole
(1990) have estimated that if all the preterm babies in British
neonatal units were fed breast milk, 100 deaths a year from
necrotising enterocolitis would be prevented.

Taking breastfeeding as the 'gold standard', bottle-feeding
has been shown to be associated with:

- increased risk of gastrointestinal infections
- increased risk of respiratory infection

- increased incidence of otitis media
- increased risk of urinary infections
- increased risk of atopic disease in families where there is a history
- increased risk of sudden infant death
- increased risk of diabetes
- reduced cognitive development
- decreased visual acuity
- reduced intelligence quotient (IQ) in preterm infants
- increased risk of necrotising enterocolitis.

See Appendix 5 (Health benefits of breastfeeding) for further reference sources.

The observed increase in the incidence of otitis media may also have a mechanical component. A 1994 report on the work of researchers at Southampton University suggested that a bottle teat occupies only the oral cavity, whereas the teat formed from the breast and nipple is sucked up into the baby's palate, encouraging the eustachian tube to open properly (Hall 1994, Thompson 1994).

Disadvantages for the mother

The disadvantages of not breastfeeding to a woman who has given birth include a doubling of the risk of osteoporotic hip fracture in later life and an increased risk of death from breast cancer under the age of 55 years. One study has suggested that the relative risk is more than doubled if parturient women do not breastfeed. As breast cancer is the commonest cancer in women, currently affecting one in eight women in the USA, a protective effect of this magnitude is potentially very important (Short 1994).

Fertility

The other major impact that not breastfeeding has on a child's mother is on her fertility. Of course a woman may become pregnant while her baby is still receiving some breast milk, but while the baby is receiving only breast milk from at least 65 minutes of suckling (or six feeds) per day, she is extremely unlikely to ovulate or menstruate, and the first menstruation is likely to be due to oestrogen withdrawal and anovulation (Short 1984). One study of well-nourished women who breastfed exclusively for 4–6 months, and who continued to breastfeed long after supplements were introduced into the baby's diet, found that they had an average of 10 months' lactational amenorrhoea and 11 months of anovulation (Lewis et al 1991). In these circumstances (full breastfeeding and amenorrhoea) the pregnancy rate is less than 2% (Consensus report 1988).

This very effective form of free contraception has huge implications globally, and still prevents more pregnancies worldwide than all other methods of contraception put together (Thapa et al 1988). Furthermore, while she is not menstruating, a woman is able to conserve iron and recover more fully from the effects of the blood lost at birth.

The economics of not breastfeeding

Economically, bottle-feeding makes no sense, either to the individual or the nation. In 1991, the cost of feeding an infant in Saskatchewan, Canada, on breastmilk substitutes for the first year of life was calculated as being between $1275 and $3055 (roughly equivalent to £600–1400) (Bergerman & Oleksyn 1991). In Massachusetts, USA, the 1992 figure was $500–1000 per year (roughly equivalent to £300–625) (Walker 1993), while in the UK, for the same year, the Joint Breastfeeding Initiative estimated that it cost £350 to feed an infant breastmilk substitutes for a year. This may be only 2% of the average UK family's income (assuming this to be about £18,000), but an equivalent amount of breastmilk substitutes consumes 12–14% of the income of the average family in the Philippines (Clavano 1981).

National costs are a product of the iatrogenic ill-health that results from not breastfeeding. In the USA, Cunningham concluded from his study of the hospitalisation patterns of a white middle-class population that, during the first 4 months of life, he would expect 77 hospital admissions for illness for every 1000 artificially fed infants. The comparable figure for breastfed infants is five admissions (cited in Walker 1993).

Otitis media, which is three to four times more common in artificially fed infants (Saarinen 1982), results in 30 million vis-

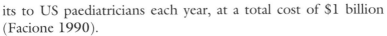

its to US paediatricians each year, at a total cost of $1 billion (Facione 1990).

In 1999, Ball & Wright published data on the excess cost of healthcare services for three illnesses (gastrointestinal, middle ear and lower respiratory infections) in the first year of life of 1000 infants, depending on whether they were artificially fed or exclusively breastfed for 3 months. After adjusting for potential confounders, they found that the bottle-fed babies made 2033 more visits to their general practitioner, required 609 more prescriptions and spent 212 more days in hospital. This cost between $331 and $475 more per never-breastfed infant (i.e. money spent to treat illnesses in babies who would not have been ill if they had been breastfed – it does not assume that breastfed babies are never ill). In the UK 200,000 of the babies born each year are never breastfed.

Regardless of socioeconomic conditions, an artificially fed baby is five times more likely to suffer from a gastrointestinal illness in the first 3 months of life. It costs around £300 per day to care for a baby in hospital. In 1991 it cost one English town £225,000 to hospitalise 150 such babies for 3–7 days each. At that rate, if 300 UK towns achieved the breastfeeding rates of Norway (90% at 3 months) or Finland (95% initiation, 75–86% at 6 months) (World Health Organisation 1990), the National Health Service would save over £67 million per year (Palmer 1993).

For each 1% increase in breastfeeding the average health authority would save £4000 in reduced hospital admissions for gastroenteritis; a 10–15% increase would thus save £40,000–60,000. The same increase in breastfeeding rates would also save the average health authority, each year, £10,000 for two cases of IDDM averted, £20,000 for four cases of neonatal necrotising entercolitis averted, and £1100 for three cases of premenopausal breast cancer averted (Woolridge 1995).

This quantifiable drain on NHS resources has resulted at last in increased government attention being paid to the subject, and money is being spent on targeting those women who are least likely to breastfeed: the young, the poor and those with the least education. However, government spending on breastfeeding is unlikely to match the huge amounts that are spent each year by those who have a vested interest in seeing breastfeeding fail. Our bottle-feeding society will turn back into a breastfeeding one only when, as a society, we see that it is in everyone's interest that children are breastfed.

Hand in hand with the acknowledgement of the overwhelming superiority of human milk for human infants will have to come a reassessment of the obstacles that are placed in the way of breastfeeding by inappropriate practices and advice. Even more importantly, but more difficult, we will have to re-acquire the skills needed to help women breastfeed successfully (described so well in *The Lancet* editorial 'A warm chain for breastfeeding' – Lancet editorial 1994).

Lactation itself is a powerful, energy-efficient survival mechanism that is not easily disturbed except by major physiological forces or by interference with its basic mechanism: appropriate suckling (Akre 1989). But breastfeeding is a learned skill. In traditional societies women learn from one another; in Western societies they are more likely to turn to health professionals, who are often ill equipped to help them.

As health professionals we also need to ask whose feelings are we protecting with the notion that women should not be made to feel guilty if they do not breastfeed: those of the women or our own? It is not inconceivable that a mother may one day sue one of the manufacturers of breastmilk substitutes (or in the dawning era of informed choice, a health professional) for not having warned her of the considerable health risks to both herself and her baby of using infant breastmilk substitutes instead of breastfeeding. Short (1994) maintains the scientific evidence for breastfeeding is now so compelling that such a mother would surely win her case.

Acknowledgement

Part of this chapter was first presented at a National Dairy Council conference and is published here with their kind permission.

References

Adler BR, Warner JO. Food intolerance in children. In: Royal College of General Practitioners Members Reference Book. London: Royal College of General Practitioners; 1991:497–502.

Akre J, ed. Lactation. In: Infant feeding – the physiological basis. WHO Bulletin 1989; 67(Suppl):23.

Arnold R et al. The psychological characteristics of infantile hypercalcemia: a preliminary investigation. Dev Med Child Neurol 1985; 27:49–59.

Aynsley-Green A. Hormones and postnatal adaptation to enteral nutrition. J Pediatr Gastroenterol Nutr 1983; 2:418–427.

Bahna SL. Milk allergy in infancy. Ann Allergy 1987; 59:131–136.

Ball TM, Wright AL. Health care costs of breastmilk substitutes feeding in the first year of life. Pediatrics 1999; 103(4):870–876.

Bergerman J, Oleksyn TA. Cited in INFACT Canada 1991; summer:2. Quoted in Walker 1993.

Brooke OG. Absorption of lard by infants. Hum Nutr Appl Nutr 39A. Cited in Minchin 1985.

Clavano RC. Assignment children. UNICEF 1981; 55/56:139–165.

Consensus report on breastfeeding as a family planning method. Lancet 1988, ii(8621):1204–1205.

Crawford MA. The role of essential fatty acids in neural development: implications for perinatal nutrition. Am J Clin Nutr 1993; 57(Suppl):703–710S.

Dallman P. Upper limits of iron in breastmilk substitutess. J Nutr 1989; 119:1852–1855.

Daniels L. Child and Antenatal Nutrition Bulletin no. 3. Health Department of Western Australia; 1989.

Dewey KG, Heineg MJ, Nommsen LA et al. Growth of breastfed and breastmilk substitutes fed infants from 0 to 18 months: the DARLING Study. Pediatrics 1992; 89(6):1035–1041.

Ebrahim GJ. Breastfeeding – the biological option. London: Macmillan; 1979.

Facione N. Otitis media: an over view of acute and chronic disease. Nurse Pract 1990; 15:11–22.

Farquharson J et al. Infant cerebral cortex phospholipid fatty-acid composition and diet. Lancet 1992; 340(8823):810–813.

Food and Chemical News. September 1980. Cited in Minchin 1985.

Hall C, ed. Health page. The Independent 1 November 1994; 25.

Hambraeus L. Proprietary milk versus human breast milk in infant feeding. Pediatr Clin North Am 1977; 24(1): 17–36.

Hernell O. The requirements and utilisation of dietary fatty acids in the newborn infant. Acta Paediatr Scand Suppl 1990; 365:20–27.

Hibbard RA, Blevins R. Palatal burn due to bottle warming in a microwave oven. Pediatrics 1988; 82:382–384.

Inch S. Breastfeeding update. In: Alexander J, Roth C, Levy V, eds. Midwifery practice core topics 3. London: Macmillan; 2000:66–83.

Jeffs SG. Hazards of scoop measurements in infant feeding. J R Coll Gen Pract 1989; 39:113.

Jelliffe DB. Unique properties of human milk. J Reprod Med 1975; 14:133.

Jelliffe DB, Jelliffe EFP. Human milk in the modern world. Oxford: Oxford Medical; 1978.

Jensen RG. The lipids of human milk. Boca Raton, FL: CRC Press; 1989.

Jones DA, West RR, Newcombe RG. Maternal characteristics associated with the duration of breastfeeding. Midwifery 1986; 2:141–146.

Joote PL et al. The effect of breastfeeding on plasma cholesterol and growth in infants. J Pediatr Gastroenterol Nutr 1991; 13: 139–142.

Karjalainen J et al. A bovine peptide as a possible trigger of insulin dependent diabetes mellitus. N Engl J Med 1992; 327:302–307.

Lancet editorial. A warm chain for breastfeeding. Lancet 1994; i(8932): 1239–1241.

Leung AKC, McArthur RG, Mc Millan DD et al. Circulating anti-diuretic hormone during labour and in the newborn. Acta Paediatr Scand 1980; 69:505–510.

Lewis PR, Brown JB, Renfree MB, Short RV. The resumption of ovulation and menstruation in a well nourished population of women breastfeeding over an extended period of time. Fertil Steril 1991; 55:529–536.

Lubec G, Wolf C, Bartosh B. Amino acid isomerisation and microwave exposure. Lancet 1989; ii(8676):1392–1393.

Lucas A, Cole TJ. Breastmilk and necrotising enterocolitis. Lancet 1990; 336:1519–1523.

Lucas A, Lockton S, Davies P. Letter. BMJ 1991; 302:351.

Lucas A, Lockton S, Davies P. Randomised trial of a ready-to-feed compared with powdered formula. Arch Dis Child 1992; 67:935–939.

Lucas A, Stafford M, Morley R et al. Efficacy and safety of LC-PUFA supplementation of infant formula milk: a randomised trial. Lancet 1999; 354:1948–1954.

Makrides M, Neumann M, Simmer K, Pater J, Gibson R. Are LC-PUFAs essential nutrients in infancy? Lancet 1995; 345:1463–1468.

Martyn T. LCPs good for business. Baby Milk Action Update 1997; 21:10.

Messenger H. Don't shoot the messenger. Health Visitor 1994; 67(5):171.

Minchin M. Breastfeeding matters: what we need to know about infant feeding. Melbourne: Alma Publications; 1985 (1st edn); 1998 (2nd edn).

Montandon CM. Breastmilk substitutes intake of one and four month old infants. J Pediatr Gastroenterol Nutr 1986; 5:434–438.

Monte CS et al. Bovine serum albumin detected in infant breastmilk substitutes is a possible trigger for insulin dependent diabetes mellitus. J Am Diet Assoc 1994; 94:314–316.

Newman J. How breastmilk protects newborns. Sci Am 1995; December:76–79.

Oski FA. Is bovine milk a health hazard? Pediatrics 1985; 75(part 2):182–186.

Palmer G. The politics of breastfeeding. London: Pandora; 1988.

Palmer G. The Mabel Liddiard Lecture, 1992: 'Who helps health professionals with breastfeeding?' Midwives Chronicle 1993; May:147–156.

Raiha NCR et al. Milk protein intake in the term infant. I. Metabolic responses and effects on growth. Acta Paediatr Scand 1986; 75(6):881–886.

Riordan J. The biological specificity of human milk. In: Riordan J, Auerbach K, eds. Breastfeeding and human lactation. London: Jones & Bartlett; 1993.

Rogan WJ. Cancer from PCBs in breastmilk? A risk benefit analysis. Pediatr Res 1989; 25:105A.

Royal College of Midwives. Comparison chart. London: RCM; 1994 (available from Royal College of Midwives, 15 Mansfield Street, London W1M 0BE; Tel: 0207 580 6523).

Saarinen UM. Prolonged breastfeeding as prophylaxis for recurrent otitis media. Acta Paediatr Scand 1982; 71:567–571.

Short RV. Breastfeeding. Sci Am 1984; 250(4):35–41.

Short RV. What the breast does for the baby, and what the baby does for the breast. Aust N Z J Obstet Gynecol 1994; 34(3):262–264.

Signman-Grant M, Bush G, Anantheswaran R. Microwave heating of infant breastmilk substitutes – a dilemma resolved. Pediatrics 1992; 90:412–415.

Sinclair CM. Fats in human milk. Topics in Breastfeeding, set IV. Victoria, NSW: Lactation Resource Centre, Nursing Mothers Association of Australia; 1992.

Slade HB, Schwartz SA. Mucosal immunity: the immunology of breast milk. J Allergy Clin Immunol 1987; 80:346–356.

Specker BL et al. Low serum calcium and high parathyroid hormone levels in neonates fed 'humanised' cows' milk based breastmilk substitutes. Am J Dis Child 1991; 145:941–945.

Stapleton T et al. The pathogenesis of idiopathic hypercalcaemia in infancy. Am J Clin Nutr 1957; 5:533–542.

Thapa S, Short RV, Potts M. Breastfeeding, birth spacing and their effects on child survival. Nature 1988; 335:679–682.

Thompson A. Doctor 1994; 27 October:23.

UNICEF, WHO, UNESCO. Facts for life – a communication challenge. 1989. Extracted in SCN News, May 1991.

Virtanen SM et al. Infant feeding in children < 7 years of age with newly diagnosed IDDM. Diabetes Care 1991; 14:415–417.

Wales JKH et al. Milk bolus obstruction secondary to the early introduction of premature baby milk breastmilk substitutes: an old problem re-emerging in a new population. Eur J Paediatr 1989; 148:676–678.

Walker B. Lead content of milk and infant breastmilk substitutes. J Food Prot 1980; 43(3):178–179.

Walker M. A fresh look at the risks of artificial infant feeding. J Hum Lact 1993; 9(2):97–107.

Watkins JB. Lipid digestion and absorption. In: Current issues in feeding the normal infant. Pediatrics 1985; 75(Suppl 1):151–156.

Weaver LT. Digestive system development and failure. In: Wilkinson AR, Tam PKH, eds. Seminars in neonatology – necrotizing enterocolitis. London: WB Saunders; 1997; 221–230.

Williams A. In: Campbell AGM, McIntosh N, eds. Forfar and Arneil's textbook of paediatrics. 4th edn. London: Churchill Livingstone; 1993:372.

Woolridge MW. Editorial. Breastmilk and premature babies. MIDIRS Midwifery Digest 1991; 1(1):5–6.

Woolridge M. Calculating the benefits of breastfeeding for purchasers and providers of healthcare. Internal document produced for UNICEF UK's Baby Friendly Initiative. London: The UK Committee for UNICEF Baby Friendly Initiative; 1995.

World Health Organization. Data bank on prevalence and duration of breastfeeding. Geneva: WHO Nutrition Unit; 1990.

Worthington-Roberts B. Human milk composition and infant growth and development. In: Worthington-Roberts B, Williams SR, eds. Nutrition in pregnancy and lactation. 5th edn. St Louis: Mosby Year Book; 1993:343.

Understanding how a baby breastfeeds

Milk production and the role of lactational hormones	23
Colostrum and milk production in the first week of life	24
Feedback inhibition of lactation	27
Milk release and infant 'sucking'	27
Changes in the breast during pregnancy and parturition	33
Variations in breast size	33

Milk production and the role of lactational hormones

Milk is produced by the glandular epithelial cells within the breast and is stored in small clusters of 'sac-like' spaces (alveoli). Around each sac is a basket array of muscle (myoepithelial) cells. Adequate milk production depends on two main factors: (1) prolactin release from the anterior pituitary, which stimulates milk manufacture, and (2) oxytocin release from the posterior pituitary, which causes the myoepithelial cells to contract, allowing the manufactured and stored milk to be released. The milk drains into the 10 to 15 'ampullae', or lactiferous sinuses, which lie behind the nipple, and removal from here is effected by the rhythmical pressure exerted by the baby's tongue (see Fig. 2.5 on p. 30). The effective functioning of both aspects of milk production is accomplished in the majority of women by means of the unrestricted and efficient suckling of the baby.

The level of prolactin in the maternal bloodstream rises steadily during pregnancy, but milk production cannot begin until the placental steroid hormones, progesterone and oestrogen, have declined (following delivery of the placenta) to the point where they no longer inhibit the action of prolactin. (Very rarely, retained placental fragments may prevent this decline (Neifert et al 1981).)

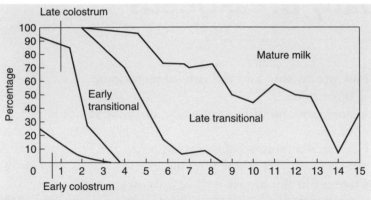

Figure 2.1 Type of milk produced during the first 2 weeks after delivery. From Humenick (1987), with permission

The length of time between placental delivery and milk synthesis varies, but seems generally to be between 48 and 96 h (Fig. 2.1).

Colostrum and milk production in the first week of life

Colostrum

Colostrum, a thick yellow fluid, begins to be synthesised in the breast from around 20 weeks' gestation. Compared with breast milk, it is particularly rich in proteins, many of which are non-nutritional, but which play an important role in gut maturation and closure.

The mother secretes very high levels of IgA in her colostrum, up to 5 mg per mL in the early days. Very little of this is absorbed, but instead remains on the surface of the baby's gut, acting as a sort of 'immunological paint' to prevent pathogens from sticking to the mucosal surfaces. Epidermal growth factor (EGF) and insulin-like growth factor (IGF) are among the most fully studied of the many growth factors and regulatory peptides found in breast milk and colostrum. EGF has been shown to accelerate maturation of the small intestinal mucosa (Weaver & Walker 1988) and strengthen the barrier properties of the gastrointestinal epithelium against digestion by endogenous and exogenous enzymes (Weaver 1997).

The prostaglandins present in human colostrum (and milk) are not digested in the infant's stomach but remain intact to protect the lining of the stomach and small intestine. Cytokines, also present, are thought to play a part in activating the infant's immune system as they also pass undigested through the stomach, and may be absorbed (Weaver 1997).

The gut of a newborn baby will allow large molecules to pass through it for some time after birth. The biological and clinical significance of this is unclear, but the timing of the first feed has a significant effect on subsequent gut permeability, which drops markedly if the first feed takes place within a few hours of birth (Vukavic 1984), implying a role for breast milk in gut closure to macromolecules (Slade & Schwartz 1987).

The giving of fluids other than the mother's colostrum/breast milk for the first 3 days of life has been shown to be associated with an increased incidence of diarrhoea in the first 6 months of life (Clemens 1999).

Although the gut of the newborn is sterile, bacteria can be detected in meconium within 4 hours of birth (Weaver & Lucas 1991).

Milk volume

There is quite a wide range in the amount of colostrum (and, later, milk) that mothers produce, but the average volume per day is quite small (see Table 2.1), certainly by comparison with the amounts an artificially fed infant may be persuaded to consume. There is no evidence that healthy term infants need fluid in any greater quantity than is made available physiologically. However, in order to receive the appropriate amount, the baby needs to be able to attach well to his mother's breast, so that he can milk the breast with his tongue. (The huge number of women who develop sore nipples while in hospital suggests that an equally large number of babies are not feeding effectively.)

In the first 3–4 hours after birth there is a major shift in water, from the intracellular to the extracellular compartments of the body, thus reducing the infant's need for fluid at this time. In addition, during the first 24 hours of life high circulating levels of antidiuretic hormone are found in the infant's blood, and this keeps urine output low (Leung et al 1980).

Milk removal

In response to appropriate stimuli, initially from suckling, nervous impulses are carried to the posterior pituitary and, by an unconditioned reflex, cause the release of oxytocin into the

Table 2.1 Milk production from birth

Age of baby	Average (range) volume per day (mL)	Average volume per feed (mL)	References
Day 1 (0–24 h)	37 (7–123)	7mls	Casey et al (1986), Houston et al (1983), Roderuck et al (1946), Saint et al (1984)
Day 2 (24–48 h)	84 (44–335)	14mls	Houston et al (1983)
Day 3 (48–72 h)	408 (98–775)	38mls	Casey et al (1986), Houston et al (1983), Neville et al (1988), Saint et al (1984)
Day 4 (72–96 h)	625 (378–876)	58mls	Houston et al (1983), Saint et al (1984)
Day 5 (96–120 h)	700 (452–876)	70mls	Casey et al (1986), Houston et al (1983), Saint et al (1984)
3 months	750 (609–837)		Butte et al (1984)
6 months	800		Neville et al (1988)

maternal bloodstream. This subsequently affects all the oxytocin receptors in the mother's body, including those in the uterus, causing the characteristic 'afterpains' often associated with early breastfeeding, particularly in multiparous women. Later, oxytocin may be released by a conditioned reflex in response to the sight or sound of the baby, or as a result of preparation for breastfeeding. There is no evidence that the *unconditioned* reflex can be inhibited by anxiety.

The 'let-down' or milk ejection reflex (in response to oxytocin release) is highly variable. In some women it is extremely vigorous, causing sharp, needle-like pains in the breast and, if the ducts are open at the nipple surface, milk may spurt out in jets. Other mothers experience a tingling sensation, and milk may only drip from the breast. At the other extreme, some mothers may experience no sensation at all, but as long as the myoepithelial cells contract sufficiently to create a positive pressure in the duct system, milk will be brought down into the lactiferous ducts where it can be stripped from the breast by the action of the baby's mouth and tongue.

This variability seems to reflect differences in maternal physiology (Lucas et al 1980), but all these responses are normal.

Once lactation is established, its continued success seems to depend rather less on high levels of prolactin, and rather more on the efficient removal of milk from the alveolar sacs. As Applebaum (1970) has said: 'Drainage, not milk production, is the sine qua non of successful breastfeeding'.

Feedback inhibition of lactation

The reason for this observation is now known to be the presence in secreted milk of a whey protein that is able to inhibit the synthesis of milk constituents (Prentice et al 1989, Wilde et al 1995). This protein accumulates in the breast as the milk accumulates and it exerts negative feedback control on the continued production of milk. Removing milk from the breast also removes the regulating protein, and milk production is stepped up again.

Efficient milk removal can be impaired, and lactation adversely affected, if the breasts are allowed to become engorged (see p. 103). In this situation the alveoli become so full that the myoepithelial cells are unable to contract strongly enough to expel the milk (Dawson 1935).

Milk release and infant 'sucking'

Milk is transferred from the breast to the baby by a combination of two processes: (1) active milk expulsion by the mother as a result of her let-down reflex, and (2) active removal by the baby who, by working on the tissues of the breast with jaw and tongue, strips milk from the milk ducts (Woolridge 1986a).

Both processes are necessary to ensure that the infant obtains both the full volume and the full nutrient content of the feed.

Much can be done to promote the first of these by encouraging the mother in her efforts to breastfeed and imbuing her with confidence in her ability to feed. This is no small task, and teaching the mother good breastfeeding technique is fundamental to these aims.

To strip the milk efficiently from the breast, both the baby and the mother will need to learn what constitutes effective attachment at the breast. The mother needs to understand how to make use of her baby's natural reflexes. To start with, the baby's entire body should be turned towards his mother and held in such a way that his neck is neither twisted nor flexed (Gunther 1973). Brushing the baby's lips against the nipple will trigger the rooting reflex (Prechtl 1958), the most important component of which is that, if encouraged correctly in the early days, the baby's mouth will gape wide to accept the breast (see Figs 2.2, 2.3 and 2.4). This contact is the only way that the young baby knows that the breast is there.

The wider the baby's gape, the easier it will be for the mother to attach her baby to her breast effectively. It is therefore important for the mother to draw a strong response from her baby in the early days (see Fig. 4.12 on p. 51).

In some cases, correct attachment may be made easier if the mother supports her breast from underneath. With a positive action, by moving her baby onto her breast, it is positioned within her baby's mouth. The mother should not push her nipple towards her baby (Fisher 1981).

The process by which the baby removes milk from the breast is analogous to hand-milking the teats of a cow's udder, whereby milk is expressed from the teat by a rhythmical rolling action of the fingers against the palm of the hand. During breastfeeding, the baby's tongue does the equivalent job of the fingers. It must be stressed that, because it is the tongue that works on the lactiferous sinuses, the relationship between these two components is crucial to good feeding (see Fig. 2.5). Consequently, locating the lower jaw well away from the base of the nipple is the first step to ensuring correct attachment (Woolridge 1986b).

The mother's nipple will extend back to the soft palate if the baby is correctly attached to the breast (see Figs 2.6 and 2.7). This stimulation of the sucking reflex (Gunther 1955, Peiper 1963) causes: (1) the baby's lower jaw to clamp on to

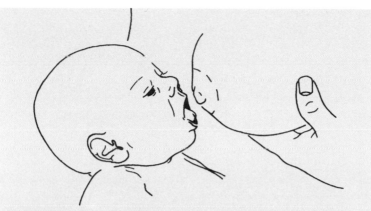

Figure 2.2

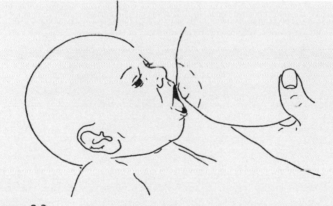

Figure 2.3

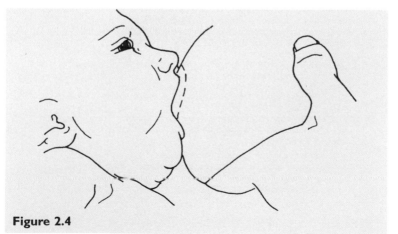

Figure 2.4

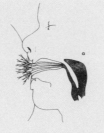

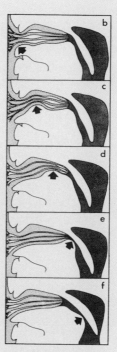

The baby is shown in median section, and exhibits good feeding technique with the nipple drawn well into the mouth, extending back to the junction of the hard and soft palate. (The lactiferous sinuses are depicted within the teat, though these cannot be visualised on scans.)

a. A 'teat' is formed from the nipple and much of the areola, with the lacteal sinuses, (which lie behind the nipple) being drawn into the mouth with the breast tissue. The soft palate is relaxed and the nasopharynx is open for breathing. The shape of the tongue at the back represents its position at rest, cupped around the tip of the nipple.

b. The suck cycle is initiated by the welling up of the anterior of the tongue. At the same time, the lower jaw, which had been momentarily relaxed (not shown) is raised to constrict the base of the nipple, thereby 'pinching off' milk within the ducts of the teat (these movements are inferred as they lie outside the sector viewed in ultrasound scans).

c. The wave of compression by the tongue, moves along the underside of the nipple in a posterior direction, pushing against the hard palate. This roller-like action squeezes milk from the nipple. The posterior position of the tongue may be depressed as milk collects in the oropharynx.

d & e. The wave of compression passes back past the tip of the nipple, in a posterior direction, pushing against the soft palate. As the tongue impinges on the soft palate the levator muscles of the palate contract, raising it to seal off the nasal cavity. Milk is pushed into the oropharynx and is swallowed if sufficient has collected.

f. The cycle of compression continues and ends at the posterior base of the tongue. Depression of the back portion of the tongue creates negative pressure, drawing the nipple and its milk contents back into the mouth. This is accompanied by a lowering of the jaw, which allows milk to flow back into the nipple.

In ultrasound scans it appears that compression by the tongue, and negative pressure with the mouth, maintain the tongue in close conformation to the nipple and palate. Events are portrayed here rather more loosely to aid clarity.

Figure 2.5 A complete 'suck' cycle

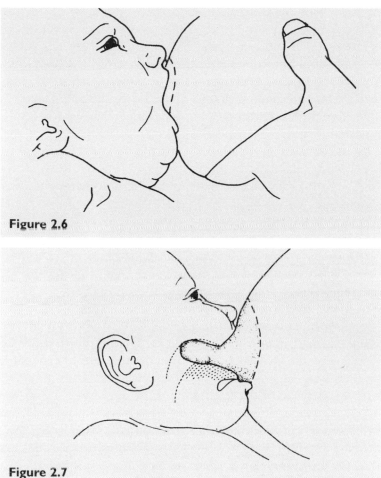

Figure 2.6

Figure 2.7

the breast tissue, (2) suction to be exerted, thus holding the nipple well into the mouth, and (3) rhythmical cycles of compression to be applied by the tongue to the teat-like shape formed from the breast and the nipple, squeezing milk from the ducts. The 'teat' lies in a furrow formed by the tongue, and the wave of compression moves back along this trough, from the breast to the baby, occluding it and forcing milk from the ampullae within the teat.

Milk will remain available for removal as long as a pressure gradient remains in the milk ducts. This is created both by positive pressure in the alveoli, due to myoepithelial contraction, and negative pressure outside the nipple, from the baby's mouth.

If the baby is attached correctly, there should be no friction of the tongue or gum on the nipple, and no movement of the breast tissue in and out of the baby's mouth. Thus the baby's sucking should not traumatise the nipple, and there should be no soreness. Pain is a biological warning signal, and in the context of breastfeeding is a sign that the feeding technique is imperfect. If this signal is not heeded, nipple damage will result. Figures 2.8 and 2.9 illustrate incorrect attachment.

Some babies appear to ingest only the milk that is ejected by the mother, taking hardly any by their own efforts. In an otherwise neurologically normal baby, this is likely to be due to early mismanagement of breastfeeding. Clinical experience suggests that, unless the baby's feeding technique is improved by better positioning, milk production will decline to below his needs.

Babies of mothers with poorly developed milk ejection must derive all their milk by actively stripping milk from the breast. For this group, correct attachment and positioning at the breast is also vital for effective milk removal.

It is worth stressing that breast milk (unlike a breastmilk substitute) is not uniform in composition. During the feed the fat (and hence the calorie) content rises as the rate of milk flow declines (see Fig. 5.1 on p. 63). This makes it very difficult to state which stage of the feed is the most nutritious. In fact the different stages are nutritious in different ways. Changes in feed management can affect the balance of nutrients taken by the baby in both the short and the long term. For this reason, arbitrary rules for breastfeeding management should not be imposed.

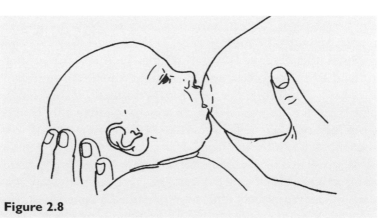

Figure 2.8

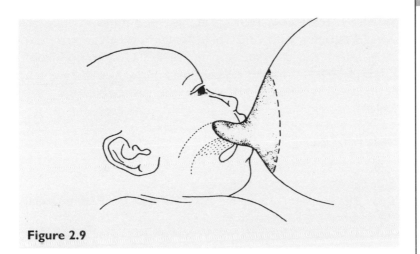

Figure 2.9

Changes in the breast during pregnancy and parturition

The changes in the breast during pregnancy are documented in most well-referenced books on the breast and breastfeeding (Neville & Neifert 1983, Vorherr 1974). As far as changes relevant to their efficiency for breastfeeding are concerned, attention has been focused in the past on the adequacy of the mother's nipples. There is little evidence to suggest that there is anything to be gained by antenatal assessment or preparation of the mother's nipples (see pp. 97–98).

The most dramatic changes in nipple shape take place around parturition and in the early postnatal period (Hytten & Baird 1958). Furthermore, with skilled help, babies can be correctly attached to breasts that may be considered to have 'inadequate nipples' (see also p. 97). There is no justification for informing a mother, on the basis of an antenatal inspection of her nipples, that she may be incapable of breastfeeding. This will serve only to damage her confidence and may be a self-fulfilling prophecy.

Variations in breast size

The size, symmetry and shape of a woman's breasts have little to do with her ability to lactate. The composition and distribution of fatty tissue in and around the lobes and fascia of the breasts varies greatly from woman to woman, but this does not influence either the composition or the volume of milk that can be **33** produced (Black et al 1998). The observed differences in milk storage capacity, which may be a function of breast size, have also shown no correlation with 24-hour milk production, although greater storage capacity may allow a mother greater flexibility with regard to her pattern of breastfeeding (Daly et al 1993).

References

Applebaum RM. The modern management of successful breastfeeding. Pediatr Clin North Am 1970; 17:203–225.

Black RF, Jarman L, Simpson JB. The science of breastfeeding. Subbury, MA: Jones & Bartlett; 1998.

Butte N, Garza C, O'Brian Smith E, Nichols BL. Human milk intake and growth in exclusively breastfed infants. J Pediatr 1984; 104:187–195.

Casey C, Neifert M, Seacat J, Neville M. Nutrient intake by breastfed infants during the first five days after birth. Am J Dis Child 1986; 140:933–936.

Daly SJ, Owens RA, Hartmann PE. The short-term synthesis and infant regulated removal of milk in lactating women. Exp Physiol 1993; 78:209–220.

Dawson EK. Edinburgh Medical Journal 1935; 42:569.

Fisher C. Breastfeeding: a midwife's view. Maternal and Child Health 1981; February:52–57.

Gunther M. Instinct and the nursing couple. Lancet 1955; i:575–578.

Gunther M. Infant feeding. Harmondsworth: Penguin; 1973.

Houston MJ, Howie P, McNeilly AS. Factors affecting the duration of breastfeeding: 1. Measurement of breastmilk intake in the first week of life. Early Hum Dev 1983; 8:49–54.

Humenick SS. The clinical significance of breastmilk maturation rates. Birth 1987; 14:175.

Hytten FE, Baird D. The development of the nipple in pregnancy. Lancet 1958; i(7032):1201–1204.

Lucas A, Drewett RF, Mitchell MD. Breastfeeding and plasma oxytocin concentrations. BMJ 1980; 281:834–835.

Neifert M, McDonough S, Neville M. Failure of lactogenesis associated with placental retention. Am J Obstet Gynecol 1981; 140:477–478.

Neville MC, Neifert MR. Lactation: physiology, nutrition and breastfeeding. New York: Plenum; 1983.

Neville M, Keller R, Seacat J et al. Studies in human lactation: milk volumes in lactating women during the onset of lactation and full lactation. Am J Clin Nutr 1988; 48:1375–1386.

Peiper A. Cerebral function in infancy and childhood. 3rd edn. New York: Consultants Bureau; 1963:418–420.

Prechtl HFR. The directed head turning response and allied movements of the human baby. Behaviour 1958; 13:212–242.

Prentice A, Addey CVP, Wilde CJ. Evidence for local feedback control of human milk secretion. Biochem Soc Trans 1989; 17:122.

Roderuck C, Williams HH, Macy IG. Metabolism of women during the reproductive years. J Nutr 1946; 32:267–283.

Saint L, Smith M, Harmann P. The yield and nutrient content of colostrum and milk from giving birth to 1 month postpartum. Br J Nutr 1984; 52:87–95.

Vorherr H. The breast: morphology, physiology and lactation. New York: Academic Press; 1974.

Vukavic T. Timing of the gut closure. J Pediatr Gastroenterol Nutr 1984; 3:700–703.

Weaver LT, Lucas A. Development of gastrointestinal function. In: Hay WW, ed. Neonatal nutrition and metabolism. St Louis: Mosby Yearbook; 1991:78.

Weaver LT, Walker WA. Epithelial growth factor and the developing human gut. Gastroenterology 1988; 94:845–847.

Wilde CJ, Addey CVP, Boddy LM, Peaker M. Autocrine regulation of milk secretion by a protein in milk. Biochem J 1995; 305:51–58.

Woolridge MW. The 'anatomy' of infant sucking. Midwifery 1986a; 2:164–171.

Woolridge MW. Aetiology of sore nipples. Midwifery 1986b; 2:172–176.

3 | Duration and frequency of feeds

Duration of feeds   36
Frequency of feeds   37
Variability in intake/infant appetite   39

Duration of feeds

In attempting to answer the question 'How long should a breastfeed last?', studies have used electronic weighing scales to seek to understand the pattern of milk transfer. Earlier work had suggested that milk transfer takes place rapidly in the first few minutes of a feed (Lucas et al 1979). This is now known to be a misleading picture derived by measuring a cross-section of babies feeding for different lengths of time. Measuring intake at repeated points during a feed has shown that such a picture does not apply to individual babies (Howie et al 1981, Woolridge et al 1982). For many mothers, milk transfer may take much longer than a few minutes, sometimes occurring very slowly. As with all biological systems there is tremendous variability in the rate at which milk is transferred from mother to baby and in the demand for milk by the baby. However, the general picture that emerges is that, if all other aspects of feeding are ideal, babies take roughly equivalent amounts of milk, but after varying periods of time on the breast (Woolridge et al 1982).

This concept is crucial to the management of breastfeeds. It suggests that babies will normally feed for a length of time that is appropriate to the rate of milk transfer, naturally regulating their intake. Thus a baby who takes milk at a high rate will feed for a short time, whereas if milk transfer occurs at a slow rate the baby will need to feed for much longer. In consequence, it is inappropriate to tell a mother how long a feed should last, and there should be no set rules on the length of feeds at any time in the postnatal period (Howie et al 1981).

However, it is important to recognise the circumstances that, if uncorrected, may cause feeds to be unnecessarily long (e.g. regularly more than 30 min per breast), as may be the case if the infant is incorrectly attached at the breast when feeding. Incorrect attachment may not only result in protracted feeds, but may cause nipple damage, the severity of which will be in direct proportion to the length of the feed. The solution in these circumstances is not to restrict the feed length (as this will create other problems; see p. 63), but to improve the attachment. Feeding can then continue without any need for restrictions.

Frequency of feeds

Initiation of breastfeeding
Healthy term newborns show signs of hunger, although the interval between feeds varies considerably, particularly during the first few days. Feeds tend to be infrequent in the first 24–48 h; as few as three feeds in the first 24 h is within the normal range and should not cause concern in an otherwise well baby. (Of 140 babies in one Japanese study, 64 fed between zero and four times in their first 24 h of life (Yamouchi & Yamanouchi 1990).) The feed frequency increases as the first week progresses, often reaching a peak around the fifth day of life (Inch & Garforth 1989) (Figs 3.1–3.3).

Range of feed frequencies from the first week onwards
The interval between feeds will determine the number of feeds the baby takes in any 24-h period. Once again, there are no set rules for either the number or the frequency of feeds that should be given. Some babies will want feeding at intervals of $1\frac{1}{2}$–2 h, whereas others will go much longer between feeds (4–6 h); mothers should be reassured that it does not matter if their baby does not appear to be 'typical'.

When breastfeeding is established, however, six to eight feeds in 24 h is the norm, and feeds that are regularly less than an hour apart may be an indication that the baby is incorrectly attached at the breast. If this is the case, the baby may be unable to consume the high-fat hindmilk. The low-fat feeds will have a rapid stomach transit time (Anonymous 1986,

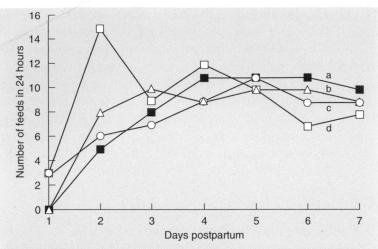

Figure 3.1 Feed frequency of four babies exclusively breastfed from birth. Adapted from Inch & Garforth (1989)

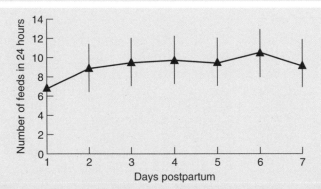

Figure 3.2 Average feed frequency of 46 breasfed babies. Adapted from Carvalho et al (1982)

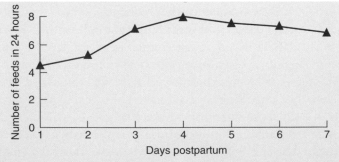

Figure 3.3 Average feed frequency of 100 breastfed babies. Adapted from Olmsted & Jackson (1950)

Spiller et al 1984) and may result in short intervals between feeds. Thus changes in management (i.e. improving feeding technique) can effect an improvement in other aspects of breastfeeding.

Variability in intake/infant appetite

Lactation is acknowledged to be regulated by the process of supply and demand, most probably with the infant's demand for milk regulating the supply (Prentice 1986, Woolridge & Baum 1987). Thus the mother of twins can produce twice as much milk as the mother of one baby, as there is twice the demand (Hartmann & Prosser 1984, Saint et al 1986) (see also p. 126–127). The amount of milk a baby 'demands' is regulated by appetite, which exerts control over the baby's intake in the same way that an adult's appetite does. This can be demonstrated by the fact that even newborn infants may finish feeding when milk is still available to them in the breast (Drewett & Woolridge 1981).

In order for the infant to regulate his intake according to his needs, he must be allowed to express his appetite fully. To do this he must: (1) be fed on demand (i.e. when he requests) and (2) be allowed to feed until satiated (i.e. for an unrestricted period of time). Only then can the natural process of appetite control operate, and the baby regulate his intake to suit his individual and changing needs. As every baby's needs differ, the pattern of feeding cannot be predicted, and should not be prescribed (Cran 1913).

Some mothers may try to restrict their baby's feeds in the belief that it is necessary (and possible) to condition him to go longer between feeds, because they cannot face the prospect of the feeding pattern of the first few weeks continuing for months. All mothers should be reassured that both the frequency and the duration of the feeds tend to decrease with time.

On the other hand, an otherwise healthy baby who is feeding less than six times in 24 h at the end of the first week may be losing his appetite. Incorrect attachment, and thus an inadequate intake, often results in apathy which is not accompanied by any other signs of illness.

References

Anonymous. Milk fat, diarrhoea and the ilial brake. Lancet 1986; i:658.

Carvalho M, Robertson S, Merkatz R, Klaus M. Milk intake and frequency of feeding in breastfed babies. Early Hum Dev 1982; 7:155–163.

Cran DHD. Breastfeeding: Dr Variot's teaching. Lancet 1913; i:1659–1660.

Drewett RF, Woolridge MW. Milk taken by human babies from the first and the second breast. Physiol Behav 1981; 26:327–329.

Hartmann PE, Prosser CG. Physiological basis of longitudinal changes in human milk yield and composition. Fed Proc 1984; 43(9):2448–2453.

Howie PW, Houston MJ, Cook A et al. How long should a breast feed last? Early Hum Dev 1981; 5:71–77.

Inch S, Garforth S. Establishing and maintaining breastfeeding. In: Chalmers I, Enkin M, Kirse M, eds. Effective care in pregnancy and childbirth. Oxford: Oxford University Press; 1989:1364–1366.

Lucas A, Lucas PJ, Baum JD. Patterns of milk flow in breastfed infants. Lancet 1979; ii:57–58.

Olmsted RW, Jackson EB. Self demand feeding in the first week of life. Pediatrics 1950; 6:396–401.

Prentice A. Cross culture differences in lactational performance. In: Hamosh M, Goldman A, eds. Human lactation 2. New York: Plenum Press; 1986.

Saint L, Maggiore P, Hartmann PE. Yield and nutrient content of milk in 8 women breastfeeding twins and 1 woman breastfeeding triplets. Br J Nutr 1986; 56:49–58.

Spiller RC, Trotman IF, Higgins BE et al. The ilial brake – inhibition of jejunal motility after ilial fat perfusion in man. Gut 1984; 25:365–374.

Woolridge MW, Baum JD. The regulation of human milk flow. In: Lindblad B, ed. Perinatal nutrition. Nutrition Symposia 1987; 6:243–257.

Woolridge MW, Baum JD, Drewett RF. Individual patterns of milk intake during breastfeeding. Early Hum Dev 1982; 7:265–272.

Yamouchi Y, Yamanouchi I. Breastfeeding frequency during the first 24 hours after birth in full term neonates. Pediatrics 1990; 86:171–175.

Correct positioning and attachment of the baby at the breast

Introduction 41
The different appearances of breast and bottle-feeding 41
When to offer help to the mother 43
Steps to achieving correct attachment 43
Indications that the baby is properly attached 49
Ways in which the midwife can help directly 51
Postural considerations 53

Introduction

A very high proportion of early breastfeeding problems may be due to a failure to attach the baby correctly to the breast. When babies are poorly attached, the mouthful of breast tissue taken in by the baby is inadequate for the jaw and tongue to express the milk effectively.

Unfortunately, many of the problems commonly associated with incorrect attachment, such as nipple pain and soreness without overt signs of infection, protracted feeds, a baby that cries hungrily after a feed and 'breastmilk insufficiency', are still reported, followed by the statement: 'The baby was properly on'. This suggests that midwives' assessment of what constitutes 'properly on' differ greatly. It is important for midwives to reassess their criteria for making this statement, for it is an issue about which there should be no complacency.

The different appearances of breast- and bottle-feeding

Industrialised Western society has become unfamiliar with the sight of a mother breastfeeding in public. As a result it may be imagined that the baby with a breast in his mouth should look much the same as a baby with a bottle teat in his mouth (Fisher 1981). This is not the case, as the 'sucking' action on the breast is mechanically different from that on the bottle (Ardran et al 1958a,b, Woolridge 1986) (see Figs 4.1 & 4.2).

As a demonstration of the difference, try this simple exercise: place a finger in your mouth as if it were a bottle teat, and suck. You will notice that your cheeks cave in as suction is created. Now suck your forearm, so that your mouth is full, as should be the case with breastfeeding. Your mouth and jaw action will be very different, involving all the muscles of your face.

An appreciation of the intrinsic, qualitative difference between breast and bottle-feeding is a necessary part of teaching good feeding technique to a mother. Commercial literature sug-

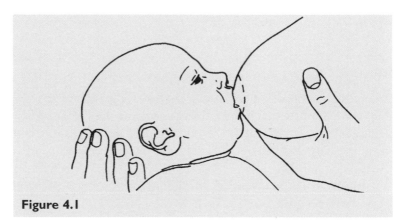

Figure 4.1

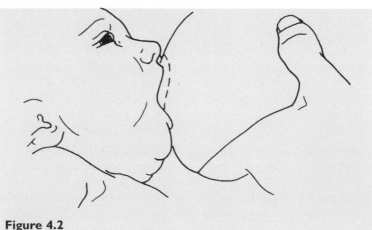

Figure 4.2

gesting that any teat is similar to the breast should be disregarded (Minchin 1998).

When to offer help to the mother

There are two different circumstances in which the guidelines offered here may be of help to midwives, and it is important to distinguish between them.

A soundly based knowledge of the physiology, together with the skills derived from close observation and familiarity with breastfeeding, should enable all midwives to provide the help and support required by mothers as they begin to breastfeed. Initially, however, this help should consist of verbal instruction only; the midwife should describe the essential features of good feeding technique to the mother and suggest possible ways in which she may improve it.

Only if a mother is unable to achieve a satisfactory feeding technique and clearly needs assistance should the midwife give more direct help. This may also apply if specific problems present themselves at a later stage, in which case the midwife may need to offer active help at this time.

It may be that, on occasions, professionals intervene too quickly, rather than observing and encouraging the mother's own efforts. However, it should be remembered that 'once the baby (and also the mother) has experienced one satisfactory feed, subsequent feeds should be better' (Gunther 1945). If the midwife feels that the 'satisfactory feed' can best be achieved with her active help, she should not be afraid to give it.

Steps to achieving correct attachment

1. Whatever the exact orientation of the baby's body relative to his mother's, he should be close to her with his head and shoulders turned towards her breast in such a way that he is square on to his mother's breast. For most mothers this will mean that the baby comes up to the breast from below, so that the baby's upper eye could make eye contact with the mother's.

   The instruction to position the baby 'chest to chest' or 'tummy to tummy' implies that the baby must be absolutely square to the mother's trunk, i.e. lying on his side. This will be helpful only if the mother is small breasted and her breasts point forward rather than down (Fig. 4.3a). However, many Western women's breasts point downwards (and outwards), which means that the baby will need to face slightly upwards and will thus be moved upwards to the breast (Fig. 4.3b).

From a side view it should be possible to draw an imaginary straight line from the centre of the base of the breast through the nipple to the centre of the back of the baby's head (see Fig. 4.3b).

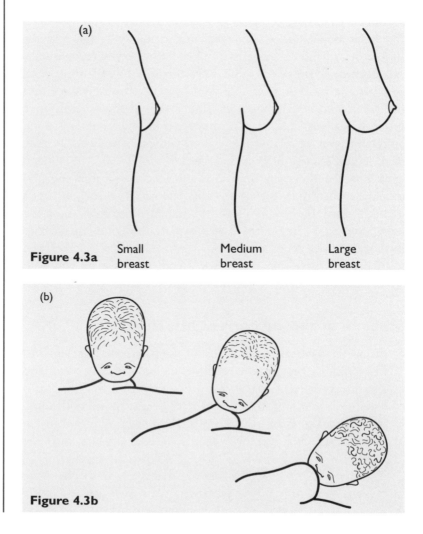

(a)

Figure 4.3a Small breast   Medium breast   Large breast

(b)

Figure 4.3b

2. The baby's head and shoulders should be supported in such a way that the head is free to extend slightly as the baby is brought to the breast, so that the chin and lower jaw reach the breast first.

3. The baby's nose and top lip should be in line with the nipple (Figs 4.4–4.7) before attempting to attach the baby. This ensures that the rooting reflex can be triggered easily by brushing the baby's mouth against the nipple.

4. Having elicited the gape, the baby (head, shoulders and trunk) should be moved straight towards the breast with a swift, positive and well-directed action. There should be no sudden change of direction such as would be the case with flexion of the head or movement away from the midline of the breast.

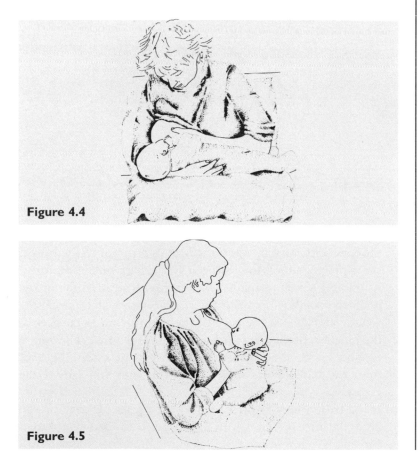

Figure 4.4

Figure 4.5

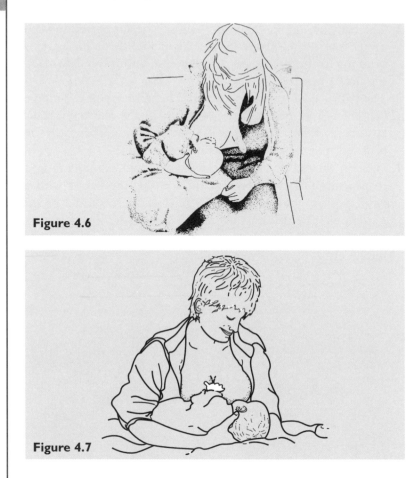

Figure 4.6

Figure 4.7

5. The lower one-third of a baby's gaping mouth is occupied by the tongue, so that if, when the baby is brought to the breast, the nipple is aimed towards the lower part of the mouth it will simply come up against the tongue. Instead, if the nipple is aimed into the upper third of the mouth it will lie along the tongue and against the roof of the mouth, and as far back as the junction of the hard and soft palate (Fig. 4.8). The baby's tongue will then lie against the breast tissue extending back from the base of the nipple, and the chin will indent the breast.

6. If the baby's nose is pressed into the breast, he may be too high on the breast, causing his neck to become flexed. Moving him lower, while still keeping him close to his moth-

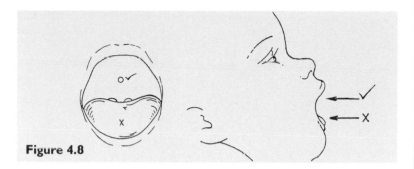

Figure 4.8

er's body, will ensure that his neck and head are extended and that his nose is free. If the baby is lying across his mother's body, his whole body may need to be moved back, feet first, towards the breast that is not being suckled. This will also have the effect of slightly extending his head and neck.

If the head and neck are slightly extended, there will be no need to press the breast away from his nostrils. Doing so tends to pull the nipple back, and may compress the milk sinuses within the breast, thus preventing milk flow. However, hyperextension of the baby's head and neck must also be avoided, as it makes swallowing impossible. If the baby's bottom lies out across the mother's lap, pulling his hips closer in towards the mother's trunk should create a space between nose and mouth.

7. Opinions differ as to which hand should be used for: (i) supporting and presenting the breast, and (ii) supporting the baby and moving him towards the breast. Mothers (and/or babies) often have a preferred side, and feeding technique may be improved on the less favoured side by using the same hands for the same tasks as on the preferred side. This may entail changing the direction in which the baby lies.

8. Many mothers and babies benefit from the breast being well supported, especially if the mother has large, soft breasts. This support can be provided either with the mother's fingers placed flat against her ribs at the base of her breast, or with her hand cupping her breast. In the latter case, her thumb should be on top of her breast, but well away from her nipple, with her remaining four fingers below (Fig. 4.9), to avoid compressing the lactiferous sinuses.

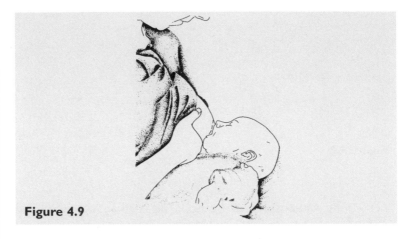

Figure 4.9

It is important that the mother is discouraged from using a 'scissor grip' when offering her breast. This pushes the glandular tissue backwards, preventing the baby from drawing the lactiferous sinuses into his mouth, and the fingers themselves prevent the baby from getting far enough on to the breast.

9. It is sometimes helpful to tilt a large or soft breast up as the baby is put on, pointing the nipple towards the roof of his mouth, or even at his nose. This helps to locate his lower lip and jaw well away from the base of the nipple.

10. When supporting her baby, the mother should either support the head and shoulders on her forearm (closer to her wrist than her elbow) (see Fig. 4.4) or hold her baby across the shoulders with her free hand, supporting his head with her fingers (see Fig. 4.7). She should be discouraged from holding the back of his head with her hand, as this may cause him distress, particularly if his head is forced on to the breast.

11. The mother should hold her baby in a position that she finds comfortable and manageable. If she is having difficulty, she might find it easier to change hands, and hold her baby with the hand opposite the breast being fed from, while she is learning. Alternatively she might like to hold her baby under her arm on the less easy side, so as to do the same job with the same hands for both breasts.

Indications that the baby is properly attached

1. If the baby is properly attached, his mouth will be wide open and the lower lip will be further away from the base of the nipple than the top lip (Fig. 4.10). With a deep mouthful of breast the bottom lip will be curled back by contact with the breast and will be some way from the base of the nipple. It is not necessary to look for this to know whether the baby is well attached. If the baby is well attached it may not be possible to see the bottom lip at all (Fig. 4.11).

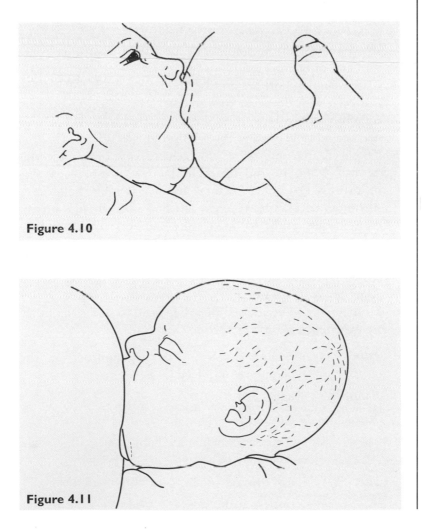

Figure 4.10

Figure 4.11

    If the lower lip appears to be pinching at the base of the nipple, the baby is not properly attached.

2. The baby will have a mouth full of breast, which will include the nipple, much of the areola and all the underlying tissue including the milk ducts. This will cause a typical jaw action as the baby works on the breast. The jaw muscles work rhythmically, and this action extends as far back as the ears. If the cheeks are being sucked inwards, the baby is not properly attached.

3. Do not be guided by how much areola can be seen above the baby's top lip, as this gives no indication as to where the tongue and the lower jaw are located. There is much variability between mothers in the size of the areola, and the advice to 'get all the areola into the baby's mouth' is irrelevant and often impractical.

4. After an initial short burst of sucking, the rhythm will be slow and even with deep jaw movements. Pauses are uncommon early in the feed once the milk has started to flow but they become more marked as the feed progresses.

5. The well-attached baby will release the breast spontaneously when he has finished the feed. A baby is able to express satiety, as well as hunger, by his behaviour. Although babies often appear satisfied after the first breast, many babies 'come to' after a few minutes. This may be a good time to change the nappy. The second breast should always be offered, unless the baby is asleep. The baby will either take the offered breast, or not, according to his appetite (see p. 64).

6. Mothers should be advised that they need to seek help if they are experiencing any of the following.

Pain	– except possibly brief discomfort at the beginning of a feed
Breasts	– engorged
Nipples	– damaged
	– compressed when the baby comes off (a white 'line' may be visible)
Baby	– not coming off the breast spontaneously
	– restless at the breast

- not satisfied after the feed
- taking a long time to feed (regularly more than 30–40 min)
- feeding very frequently (i.e. more than 10 feeds in 24 h)
- feeding very infrequently (i.e. fewer than three feeds in the first 24 h or fewer than six feeds in 24 h at 24–48 h old)
- still passing meconium at 36–48 h.

Ways in which the midwife can help directly

One of the most important things you should do is to describe what you are doing, and why you are doing it.

1. Hold the baby behind his shoulders with the heel of your hand, and with your fingers supporting the base of his head.
2. It may be helpful, when the breast is large or soft, to 'firm' it by applying gentle pressure with the other hand, placing your thumb below and your fingers on top.
3. Move the baby against the breast, teasing him by brushing his upper lip against the nipple. Wait until he begins to open his mouth wide before moving him on to the breast.
4. When you are confident that he will open his mouth widely, and the moment that you see the lower lip start to drop, move him on to the breast quickly with a positive but gentle action (Fig. 4.12).

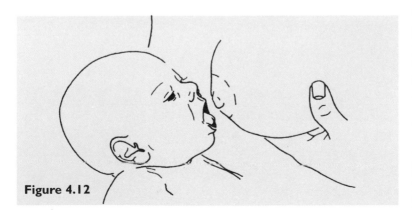

Figure 4.12

5. Aim the baby's bottom jaw as far away from the base of the nipple as possible, so that he gets as much of the breast in his mouth as he can. He must get far enough on to the breast so that he can squeeze milk out of the ducts behind the areola with his tongue (Fig. 4.13). Do not tip his head forward, but move the whole baby towards the mother, keeping his spine straight and his head slightly extended.

6. It is the baby's lower jaw and tongue that work at the breast, so less of the areola will be visible below the lower lip than above the top lip, and his mouth will appear asymmetrically placed (Fig. 4.14). When you are helping the mother in this way, tell her what you are doing and why, and she will then be more likely to achieve it herself.

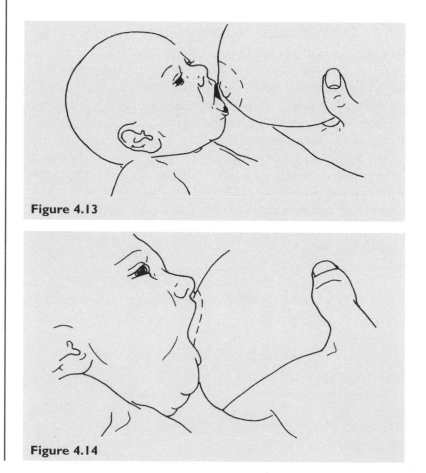

Figure 4.13

Figure 4.14

Many mothers use forceful terms to describe the way in which their baby was handled by helpers, for example: 'My baby was "rammed" on to my breast'. It is wholly inappropriate to force the baby on to the breast; rather he should be enticed to respond to the breast. Pressure on the back of the baby's head can be very distressing to both mother and baby. A sensitive hold and skilled timing are the hallmarks of good practice.

Postural considerations

Suggestions for the first feed

The mother's physical comfort when breastfeeding is important. She may be inclined to overlook any personal discomfort while focusing her attention on the needs of her baby.

Before assisting the mother with the feed it may be appropriate to offer a bed pan, a fresh sanitary pad or more general toileting. The midwife should explain the importance of being comfortable for this and all subsequent feeds.

Such preparation should be made in good time, before the baby is crying hungrily for a feed, as a crying baby cannot easily take the breast. Similarly, the mother should be told that it is not essential to change her baby's nappy before he goes to the breast. (A baby should never be allowed to become distressed before the breast is offered.)

The mother may have definite views about the position she wishes to adopt for feeding, and this must be respected. However, positions that are appropriate for later feeding sessions may not be so for the early feeds, particularly if the mother has perineal or abdominal sutures, or has received an epidural or spinal anaesthetic.

The following position for feeding is described in detail, as it is likely to be comfortable for the mother, baby and midwife, particularly for the first few feeds.

Helping the mother to feed lying down

This position is a useful one in which to help the mother. The difficulty with it for the mother is that she may be unable to use the arm on which she is lying to help put her baby to the breast. She should be encouraged to use her free hand to bring her baby towards her, rather than use it to try to put her breast into his mouth (Fig. 4.15).

The midwife should recognise that she probably has a preference for helping on one particular side, and unless the mother needs specific help with one breast she should opt for that side. The midwife may be able to use the same hand to help to feed the baby from the other breast if she raises the baby on a pillow and asks the mother to roll slightly towards her baby. The midwife may have only one or two opportunities to help a particular woman. The more competent she is, the more confidence she will give the mother (Fig. 4.16).

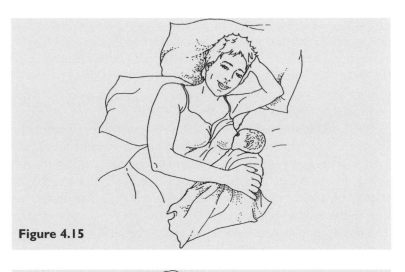

Figure 4.15

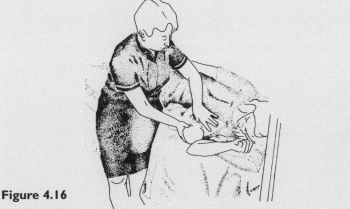

Figure 4.16

It should be suggested to the mother that she lie on her side, with her head supported by pillows. If lying on her left side, her left arm should be flexed, with her forearm parallel with her head. She may need a pillow in the small of her back, and one between her knees, for added comfort and support.

Raising the mother's chest with the short edge of the pillow will bring the breast further away from the mattress; this may make good attachment of her baby easier.

The baby should be placed beside and facing his mother, so that he can see her face. He should not be wrapped in a blanket, so that his hands and feet can make contact with her. The bedclothes should be tucked loosely round the baby and under the mattress, to ensure warmth and safety.

Allow time for the mother and her baby to interact. The mother may talk to and stroke her baby, or give him her finger to hold. The baby's rooting reflex may be stimulated by the tactile and olfactory sensations he receives.

The mother may comment that her baby appears hungry, but if she does not the midwife should indicate to her that her baby seems ready to feed.

The baby should be guided gently towards the breast and the mother helped, if necessary, to attach him correctly to the breast (see p. 51).

If the midwife has helped to attach the baby, the mother should be encouraged to place her free hand where the midwife's was, once the baby is correctly attached. Provided the safety of the mother and baby is assured, the midwife can then withdraw a little, unless the mother needs further help, for example to put her baby to the other breast (Fig. 4.17).

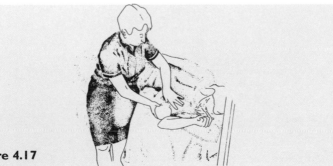

Figure 4.17

If the mother experiences correct attachment at the first feed, it is unlikely that she will tolerate incorrect attachment at later feeds. While the mother's and baby's bodily positions may change from feed to feed, the technique of attachment remains the same. This needs to be made clear to the mother.

Helping the mother to feed sitting up

In most Western societies, the traditional position for breastfeeding has been sitting upright on a nursing chair. Such chairs were of an appropriate height and had no arm rests. However, modern furniture does not always lend itself to good breastfeeding positioning. Often it is too soft, has obstructive armrests and/or sloping backs. Hospital beds and backrests which encourage the mother to lean back are similarly unhelpful.

To achieve correct positioning of the baby at the breast while seated, the mother should be encouraged to lean forwards slightly, so that her breast also falls forward, facilitating attachment. Leaning back flattens the breast, making it much more difficult.

She may need additional pillows to support her back or arms, or raise her baby to a more comfortable level (Figs 4.18 & 4.19).

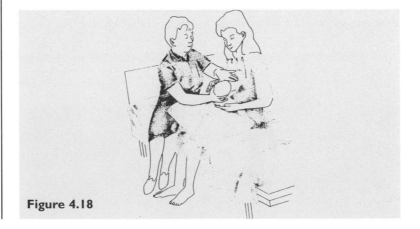

Figure 4.18

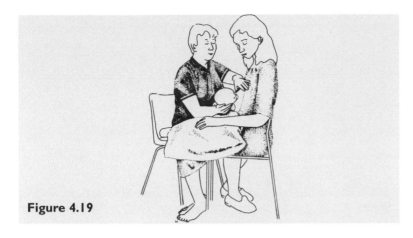

Figure 4.19

Having attached her baby correctly, the mother can then be encouraged to relax her back and shoulders against the supporting chair. A footstool may also be a useful aid to relaxation, but her knees should be only very slightly higher than her hips so that her lap is almost flat. Her feet should also be flat, on either the floor or the footrest.

Position and posture of the midwife
Many midwives experience backache and other discomforts when assisting mothers with breastfeeding. It is important that midwives consider their own comfort as well as that of the mother, and avoid positions that will put undue strain on their muscles (Figs 4.20–4.22).

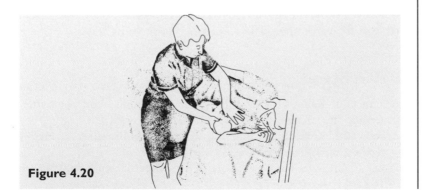

Figure 4.20

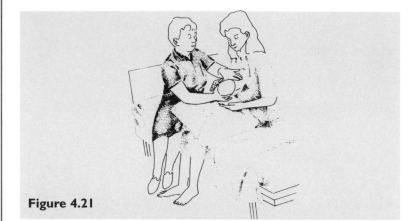

Figure 4.21

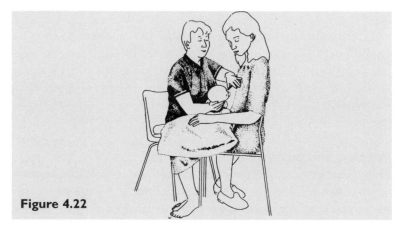

Figure 4.22

The midwife will find it helpful to keep one foot on the floor if she is sitting on the side of the bed (Fig. 4.21). If she needs to lean forwards she should keep her back straight.

References

Ardran GM, Kemp FH, Lind J. A cineradiographic study of bottle-feeding. Br J Radiol 1958a; 31:11–22.

Ardran GM, Kemp FH, Lind J. A cineradiographic study of breast-feeding. Br J Radiol 1958b; 31:156–162.

Fisher C. Breastfeeding: a midwife's view. Maternal and Child Health 1981; February:52–57.

Gunther M. Sore nipples: causes and prevention. Lancet 1945; ii:590–593.

Minchin M. Breastfeeding matters: what we need to know about infant feeding. Melbourne: Alma Publications; 1998.

Woolridge MW. The 'anatomy' of infant sucking. Midwifery 1986; 2:164–171.

5 Factors that have been shown to help

Advice and support at the first feed   60
Unrestricted feeds   63
Feeding the baby at night   66
Monitoring the baby's health and well-being   69

Advice and support at the first feed

The psychological impact on the mother of her first breastfeeding experiences is of undoubted importance. A woman who has just given birth will attach great significance to the way her baby reacts to her, and this may affect her feelings towards her baby. A successful first feed is likely to make the mother feel that her baby likes her, and this may be crucial to the continuance of breastfeeding in either the short or the long term (De Chateau 1980).

In the past, midwives encouraged suckling soon after the birth, because they recognised the benefit with regard to physiological placental delivery. Successive surveys by the Office of Population Censuses and Surveys (OPCS) (White et al 1992) and the Office of National Statistics survey (Foster et al 1997) have shown that the early initiation of breastfeeding is associated with a longer duration of breastfeeding. This association is supported by controlled studies.

Researchers in Dundee (Salariya et al 1978) randomly assigned mothers to different breastfeeding regimens relating to the timing of the first and subsequent feeds. The mothers were followed for 18 months, at which time the researchers were able to conclude that babies who were first fed within 30 min of birth were likely to remain breastfed for longer. Smaller controlled studies in the United States (Winters 1973), Sweden (De Chateau & Wiberg 1977) and Canada (Thomsen et al 1979), which combined early contact and early suckling, support these findings. They also noted that early contact positively affected the behaviour of mothers towards their babies.

Although the benefits of early feeding and early contact have been well documented, controversy still exists as to whether it is the early contact per se or the early suckling that contributes to the extended feeding period. A study conducted in Thailand (Woolridge et al 1985) suggested that the quality of the contact may also be important. Mothers who have been separated from their babies soon after delivery should be reassured that high-quality contact may be equally valuable whenever it is offered.

It is the midwife's responsibility to ensure that each mother has a satisfactory first feed, as soon as both mother and baby are ready. All mothers should be encouraged to hold their babies with skin-to-skin contact within 30 min of a normal birth. In most cases the baby will be ready to feed (as distinct from other forms of close contact) within the first hour after birth (Widstrom et al 1987). Yet in observations of labour ward practices, carried out in eight health districts in England as part of the 'policy and practice in midwifery' study (Garforth & Garcia 1987), researchers found that the average time that elapsed between a normal birth and the first feed was 98 min; which suggests that some feeds were being delayed unnecessarily. Furthermore they found that in only 44% of cases was a midwife involved with the feed.

Even though the standard delivery bed is not designed to accommodate more than one person, infants may safely experience their first feed while still in the delivery room, provided reasonable care is taken and delivery staff are skilled in helping.

Breastfeeding is a skill to be learned and practised. Many first-time mothers have never seen anyone breastfeeding, and although breastfeeding is natural it is not instinctive (Gunther 1955). Even multiparous women may need help to get started, particularly if they have never breastfed before, or have had previous difficulties. It is the midwife's responsibility to impart the necessary information about breastfeeding, but whether this is done at the first feed or later as an integral part of the mother's postnatal education must be decided on an individual basis.

The psychological component of successful breastfeeding should not be underestimated. Midwives, in their supporting role as breastfeeding experts, should reassure the mother that her breasts and nipples are anatomically suitable for the purpose of breastfeeding (unless this is inappropriate) and reinforce her success with praise.

It is hoped that midwives will develop a standardised policy within their workplace in line with the Ten Steps to Successful Breastfeeding (see Appendix 1) in relation to giving essential breastfeeding information and, where appropriate, offering breast-feeding instruction and advice. A policy exists in most health authorities to ensure that all bottle-feeding mothers are instructed individually in the making up of formula feeds and the sterilisation of bottles. The giving of breastfeeding advice should also be regarded as an integral part of the midwife's responsibility for postnatal education, and should be given equal priority.

Appropriate teaching at the first or later feeds should include some or all of the following information.

- The composition of colostrum and mature milk should be explained to the mother, who will then understand why her breastfed baby does not require the large volumes given to bottle-fed babies in the first few days of life. She can be informed that colostrum is unique and meets her newborn baby's requirements completely, provided her baby has unre-stricted access to the breast.
- From the very first feed the mother needs to know the importance of correct attachment, as well as being shown how to achieve it.
- The physiology of lactation needs to be outlined, using the feed itself to explain: (1) the 'let down' of milk, and (2) the mechanism of milk removal. Explaining the baby's sucking rhythm helps the mother to understand that the pauses are an integral part of the feed and that there is no need to stimulate her baby to suck continuously.
- The mother will need to know about her baby's probable feeding needs during the early postnatal period. Information concerning the variable composition of the milk he will receive during a feed (i.e. the graded change from foremilk to hindmilk) will help her to appreciate that she should not attempt to restrict the duration of his feeds.
- She should also be told that there may be periods, as her baby grows, when his feeding frequency may increase for a day or so. It is thought that this is the baby's way of ensuring that the milk supply remains adequate for his increasing needs.

Unrestricted feeds

Unrestricted duration of feeds

For many years there has been a widespread belief that it was necessary to limit sucking time, particularly in the early days, in order to prevent sore nipples (King 1913, Naish 1913, Liddiard 1924–1948) (see also Ch. 8, Prevention of feeding problems). Several studies have shown that nipple soreness is not affected by the duration of the feed (Carvalho et al 1984, Slaven & Harvey 1981).

Unfortunately the advice to a mother to limit her baby's suckling time, at either or both breast(s), will not only do no good, it will in many cases do harm (Kries et al 1987, Woolridge & Fisher 1988). It has been known for some time that the composition and rate of flow of milk from the human breast changes as the feed progresses (Hytten 1954). The result is that at the start of the feed the baby takes a large volume of lower-calorie milk (foremilk), which gradually increases in fat and decreases in volume as the feed progresses (hindmilk) (Hall 1975) (see Fig. 5.1).

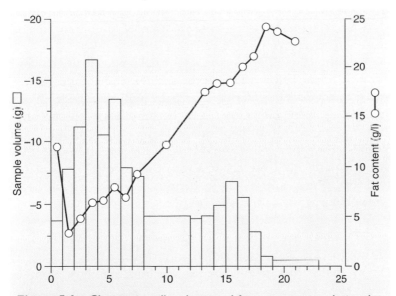

Figure 5.1 Changes in milk volume and fat concentration during the course of a feed on one breast. Reproduced with permission from Woolridge M, Fisher C. Colic, 'overfeeding' and symptoms of lactose malabsorption in the breastfeeding : a possible artefact of feed management? Lancet 1988; ii: 382–384. © by the Lancet Ltd.

It has also been shown that babies will feed at the breast for very different lengths of time if left undisturbed, and that the length of the feed is probably determined by the rate of milk transfer between mother and baby (Woolridge et al 1982) (see p. 12). Thus, although there are many babies who will terminate a feed spontaneously in under 10 min, those who have a slow rate of transfer will take longer than this. Even though they may not be consuming large volumes after this time, the milk may be sufficiently high in fat (and therefore calories) to make a significant contribution to the energy value of the feed (contrary to what has been shown by Lucas et al 1979). If the mother believes that she must limit her baby's time at the breast, or that she must use both breasts at each feed (and therefore deliberately removes him from the first breast before he finishes spontaneously), she may be significantly curtailing her baby's calorie intake. In such situations the baby may fail to gain weight despite frequent feeds and an apparently good supply of milk (Fisher 1987).

Overproduction of milk, causing discomfort and distress, may also be a consequence of limiting feeds, as the baby seeks to compensate for his reduced calorie intake by feeding more frequently, thereby removing large amounts of foremilk which are rapidly replaced (Woolridge & Fisher 1988).

A mother should be encouraged to allow her baby to finish the first breast before offering the second, and should be reassured that it does not matter if her baby wants to feed from only one breast at an individual feed. If she starts with the other breast at the next feed there should be no long-term imbalance in milk production. She should be similarly reassured that if her baby requires both breasts at a feed this is equally acceptable, and that he may shift from one pattern of feeding to another as the volume of milk adjusts to his needs.

Unless the total duration of the feed is very protracted (see p. 37), which may indicate that the mother needs more help to ensure that her baby is attached correctly, the baby is likely to 'know' better than anyone else for how long (and how often) he needs to be fed.

Unrestricted frequency of feeds

It has already been noted that the steadily increasing number of women delivered in hospital received the misguided advice that they should regulate the frequency of their baby's feeds. Gradually, however, careful observations of the unrestricted feeding behaviour of normal infants were made and published (Olmsted & Jackson 1950, Simsarian & McLendon 1942, 1945). It became apparent from these and later studies (Carvalho et al 1984, 1982) that feeds are usually infrequent for the first day or so, rapidly increase between the third and seventh day, and then decrease (see p. 38). It was also found that, although some babies with frequencies at the lower end of the scale were content to feed only six times in 24 h, the vast majority required feeding more frequently than this, especially after the first few days. Observational studies also revealed that the intervals between feeds, for the first few weeks of life at least, were unpredictable, appearing random, ranging from 1 to 8 h.

Subsequently, evidence has accumulated to suggest that babies who are allowed to regulate the frequency of their feeds themselves gain weight more quickly (Illingworth & Stone 1952, Salver 1956) and remain breastfed for longer (Illingworth & Stone 1952, Martin & Monk 1982) than those who have arbitrary rules imposed on them. The evidence provided by such research has formed the basis for the gradual adoption in most maternity units (Martin & Monk 1982) of the more physiological and beneficial practice of demand, or baby-led, feeding, which simply consists of feeding the baby whenever he wishes and for as long as he wishes. (See Step 8 of the Ten Steps, Appendix 1.)

Midwives may find, however, that they are caring for breastfeeding women who are still under the mistaken impression that regular, 4-hourly feeding is the normal pattern of behaviour for the majority of breastfed newborn babies. This belief will serve only to undermine confidence in their ability to breastfeed their babies satisfactorily on their breast milk alone, when they find, as the majority will, that their own babies need feeding more frequently than this. A simple explanation of the physiology of lactation and the value of baby-led feeding, both to the baby (reducing the incidence of jaundice (see p. 79) and improving weight gain (Illingowrth & Stone 1952, Salver 1956)) and to the mother (in establishing successful lactation (Illingworth & Stone 1952) and preventing engorgement (see p. 103)) may need to be incorporated sensitively into the early physical assistance that the midwife provides.

Feeding the baby at night

The value of night feeds

Milk production continues as efficiently at night as by day, and if the milk is not removed as it is formed (as regulated by the baby's need to go to the breast) the volume of milk in the breast will rapidly exceed the capacity of the alveoli. The consequent engorgement is not only uncomfortable for the mother, but it will begin the process of lactation suppression (see p. 27). Feeding the baby at night will minimise or prevent the potential problem of engorgement (see p. 103).

Once lactation is established, night feeds provide the infant with a substantial proportion of his 24-h intake. The younger the baby, the more likely he is to consume the same volume of milk during the 12 h from 5pm and 5am as between 5am and 5pm (i.e. 50% on average) (Dewey & Lonnerdal 1983). It is therefore to be expected that the baby will be hungry at night, and assuaging this hunger with formula feeds may lead to lactation suppression in the mother.

Although the long-term relationship between prolactin levels and milk production has not been clearly defined (Glasier et al 1984), it does appear that high levels of prolactin are necessary not only for the initiation of lactation, but are directly related to milk yields in the first 2 weeks at least (Aono et al 1982, Kauppila et al 1981, Ylikorkala et al 1982). It has also been demonstrated that prolactin release in response to night-time suckling is greater than during the day; thus milk production may get its greatest 'boost' when the baby feeds at night (Glasier et al 1984, Howie 1985).

As prolactin levels have been shown to rise in response to suckling, the practice of baby-led feeding is likely to result in higher basal prolactin levels. The frequent suckling, which results in increased prolactin levels, also suppresses ovulation, although the exact mechanism is not yet clear (Howie 1985).

The contraceptive effect of breastfeeding, although not 100% reliable, may be of great importance to those who for personal or religious reasons do not wish to use conventional (Western) methods, and it is therefore vital that these women are not subjected to any restrictions on feeds, especially at night[a].

It is often thought to be a kindness to the newly delivered woman to remove her baby from her bedside so that she can sleep. However, the baby will probably sleep for quite a long time after his post-delivery alertness (Simsarian & McLendon 1942, Macfarlane 1977). During this time his mother can also sleep if she wishes.

Subsequently the mother needs to be able to put her baby to her breast during the night, not only to encourage lactation (Krnjevic & Phillis 1963, McNeilly et al 1983), but to 'practise' attaching her baby to the breasts while they are still soft, in preparation for effective milk removal. Furthermore a woman delivered in hospital needs to have experienced her baby's feeding patterns 'round the clock' (Step 7 of the Ten Steps; see Appendix 1) so that she does not feel that there are any confidence-sapping gaps in her knowledge when she goes home. This information is especially valuable to primiparous women, given the current practice of short hospital stays. (Women delivered at home will acquire this knowledge automatically.)

Rooming in

A mother is more likely to sleep soundly in hospital if she has her baby beside her, as she will be confident that, if her own baby wakes, she will hear him. She is then less likely to be disturbed by the sound of other babies in the night. (This practice is advocated by Step 7 of the Ten Steps; see Appendix 1.)

Bedding-in

In many cultures the most usual place for a baby to be, night or day, is with his mother (e.g. Liedloff 1975). Indeed in some

---

a   Used correctly, the Lactational Amenorrhoea Method (or LAM) is as effective a method of contraception as the combined contraceptive pill, for the first 6 months following birth (Kennedy 1989). To be effective the baby must be less than 6 months old, fully breastfed with no restrictions of feed interval and with no long gaps between feeds. The mother must be amenorrhoeic.

societies it would be unsafe for the baby to be anywhere else. In many places the practice is so firmly entrenched that even where women give birth in hospital (e.g. Bombay in India, or Chiang Mai in Thailand) it is expected that the baby will sleep with his mother; some hospitals do not even provide cots (Anand 1981, Woolridge et al 1985).

The idea that babies 'should' sleep separately is a fairly recent feature of Western civilisation; in the mid-nineteenth century Western medical textbooks were still advocating that mother and baby should sleep together, in part to protect the baby from cold (Coombe 1840).

'Bedding-in' has apparently become less common in Western society. Health professionals seem to fear that a baby who shares his mother's bed is at risk, either from falling out of bed or from suffocation. The fears have been greatly exaggerated. Cot deaths, which by comparison are much more common, were in the past thought to be the result of overlaying. There is no evidence, today, to say categorically that bedding-in either increases or decreases the incidence of cot death (J Reed, personal communication, 1987).

In the Nair Charitable Hospital in Bombay, for example, where bedding-in is common, and has been for many years, there have been no 'accidents' as a result of babies sharing their mother's bed (Anand 1981). Although the actual number of babies who sleep with their mothers in Britain is unknown, it is undoubtedly more common at home (co-sleeping) than in hospital.

OPCS records (1985) show that accidental mechanical suffocation of a baby whilst in its parents' bed is a very rare event. Furthermore the same small number of babies died (in the same year) in their own bed or cradle as died in their parents' bed[b].

As time-lapse film has demonstrated, a healthy baby sleeping with healthy parents moves many times during his periods of sleep, adapting his position to that of his parents, and is usually in no danger of suffocating. It should, however, be stressed that both baby and parents were well; if either parent were ill, sedat-

---

b   In 1985 the total number of deaths of babies between birth and 1 year was 6141. Of these, six babies died (in their first year) from accidental mechanical suffocation, four in their parents' bed and two in their own bed or cradle (a further 1165 died as a result of cot death) (OPCS 1985).

ed, intoxicated or grossly obese, or if the baby were immobilised in plaster, bedding-in might not be advisable. In addition, the type of bedding must be considered, as very soft bedding, quilts or water beds may increase the risk to the baby (Bass et al 1986).

Recent studies suggest that co-sleeping appears to carry risk only for those parents who smoke (Fleming et al 1996).

Various solutions are available to those who fear that the baby may fall out of the bed, despite the presence of his mother. They could both sleep on a mattress on the floor; the bed could have cot-sides attached; it could be pushed up against the wall; or the bedclothes could be firmly tucked around the couple and under the mattress.

Not all mothers wish to sleep with their infants, but there seems to be no reason why those who choose to do so should be dissuaded from following their own inclinations, either in hospital or at home.

The mother's sleep

Sleep is important to the mother of a young baby, and she may be less disturbed if she uses thicker or more absorbent nappies and does not change her baby at night unless the outer clothes are wet or the baby is fretful. Minimal disturbance of a baby who has wakened only to be fed may result in the baby settling more quickly after the feed. It may also help the baby to begin to adapt to differences between day and night

The quality of sleep the newly delivered mother experiences may be improved by breastfeeding at night. Although there is no direct experimental evidence to suggest a role for oxytocin in the control of cortical activity (Paisley & Summerlee 1984), there is a suggestion that dopamine receptors in the brain mediate sedation and sleep (Corsini 1977) and that dopamine may be involved in the mechanism of oxytocin release (Clark et al 1979). If this is the case, it may account for the often reported and observed (Bourne 1983) sleepiness that many women experience when they breastfeed, which facilitates a rapid return to sleep at night (Urnas-Moberg 1989).

Monitoring the baby's health and well-being

The midwife has responsibilities for the baby, as well as for the mother in her care. This is particularly apparent when the mother and baby go home from hospital and the midwife must monitor the baby's progress for a statutory period. However, not all aspects of the health and well-being of a baby can be assessed in relation to a set of standard values. It is neither easy nor desirable to implement rigid criteria for weight gain, stool frequency and appearance, or the baby's general state of vitality, as it is for serum bilirubin or blood glucose levels.

Weight

In the short period after birth for which the midwife attends the mother and baby, it is not possible to establish whether the baby is 'on target' for his genetically determined growth trajectory. The size of the baby at birth, determined largely by placental sufficiency, will not necessarily match this later 'biological size', and there may be a variable period after birth until the balance between these two is reached.

In practice, the simplest and most readily applied 'yardstick' is that the baby should have regained his birthweight by 10 days of age, as an indication that the postnatal physiological losses have been made up. This presupposes that the baby's birth-weight was accurately measured and recorded. It should also be borne in mind that there are limitations to the accuracy of mid-wives' scales (Culley et al 1979, Whitfield et al 1981), and also that the normal daily variability in the baby's weight will make it difficult to establish the absolute weight with any certainty.

It is often assumed that it is acceptable for a baby to lose up to 10% of his birthweight. Although this was common at a time when breastfeeding frequency and duration was severely restrict-ed, there is no reason to suppose that this is normal.

It is important to realise that the midwife may influence the mother's expectations about her baby's future growth. If the information that she gives the mother is not soundly based, con-flict will be created when the mother and baby pass from her care to that of the health visitor.

Weight gain

The appropriateness of applying growth standards derived some years ago from infants who were largely formula fed, and whose intake may have been altered by imposed feeding schedules, to the exclusively breastfed baby has been questioned for some time (Whitehead & Paul 1985). Initially, the typical breastfed baby grows rapidly, gaining weight faster than a bottle-fed baby over the first 2–3 months. The rate of gain then slows at around 4 months, ultimately falling below that of the bottle-fed baby at around 6–12 months. Although previously interpreted as 'growth faltering' due to breast milk inadequacy, this pattern is now gaining acceptance as the normal one for a breastfed infant (Wood et al 1988, World Health Organization 1994).

The actual growth pattern can be determined only by routine monthly weight measurements. Measuring growth reliably over shorter periods (e.g. a week) is much more difficult, particularly in the first 2 weeks after birth when changes in weight are so dramatic and variable. However, the net gain over birthweight in the first fortnight, as estimated from neonatal growth charts (Gardner & Pearson 1971), is likely to be of the order of 100 g; roughly 20 g per day.

Weight variations

A baby's weight may fluctuate with incidental events such as passing a stool or urine or taking a feed.

In the first few days the infant will pass meconium and lose some water by evaporation. As the breastfed baby is adapted to taking only small amounts of fluid for the first few days, a net loss of weight would be expected.

It is not possible to abolish day-to-day variations when monitoring weight, but they can be reduced to a minimum by standardising the times and procedure for measuring weight (e.g. naked weight, before a feed and at the same time of day). If the baby is weighed at set intervals, preferably on the same scales each time, the general trend over time should provide useful information.

However, if conditions are not standardised, or if the baby is weighed too frequently, incidental changes such as a breastfeed (of, say 150 g) or the passage of a stool and urine (say, 180 g) will entirely swamp the anticipated daily weight increment cited above (i.e. 20 g per day).

Although it would be appropriate for the midwife to be concerned if a baby was gaining weight more slowly than expected, she should be aware that expressing too much anxiety in the mother's presence may be counterproductive. It may have the effect of damaging the mother's confidence in her ability to breastfeed.

The issue of whether the infant subsequently showed a satisfactory weight gain would have to be considered in relation to other factors, such as parental stature or gestational age, in order to assess the anticipated growth pattern of the infant in question.

Stools

The passage of the first stool by the newborn is usually indicative of a patent intestinal tract, and this fact is noted in most hospital and community settings today. The length of time taken for meconium to change to the yellow stool of the milk-fed neonate will vary according to gestational age, feeding method and pattern of feeds, and can give some indication of the baby's well-being in relation to his milk intake (Salariya & Robertson 1993).

Initially the stools of a breastfed baby vary in number and amount, and depend on the intake of colostrum. Breast milk, a complete food, is fully utilised, and the baby's stools may appear quite loose on or around the third to fifth days of life. This corresponds with the mother's milk 'coming in' and is quite normal. Thereafter the mother should be advised that her baby will continue to have quite loose stools for as long as he remains exclusively breastfed.

Breastfed babies' bowels do not necessarily move daily or at regular intervals and, provided the baby is well and the abdomen is soft, there should be no cause for concern. The stools of a breastfed baby differ from those of an artificially fed baby in several respects. They will take longer to change from black to yellow but should nevertheless be starting to change by 48 h, and should be yellow by 72–96 h if the baby has been well attached and feeding well (Salariya & Robertson 1993). The stools are much less bulky than those of an artificially fed baby and the frequency may range from once a feed to once every 12 days (Morley et al 1977, Weaver et al 1988). No intervention is necessary and the baby is not constipated, as is often suggested. It is unnecessary and unacceptable to give a breastfed baby sugary drinks (see pp. 80–83, and Appendix 1, Step 6).

The following is offered as a guide to the stool colour change expected in a healthy term infant (Fig. 5.2).

Figure 5.2 Stool colour comparator, developed at the Midwifery Department, Ninewells Hospital, Dundee, UK. Reproduced with permission

Birth – 24 hours	=	1st day meconium
24–48 hours	=	2nd day meconium/changing
48–72 hours	=	3rd day changing/yellow
72–96 hours	=	4th day yellow

A term baby who is still passing meconium at 4–5 days is probably getting insufficient milk for his needs and losing weight. Similarly, stools described as 'changing' at 4–5 days could indicate some shortcoming in relation to breastfeeding procedure, such as incorrect attachment or restricting the duration or the frequency of feeds (Salariya & Robertson 1993).

General health

Weight gain is only one of a number of indications that the newborn infant is healthy and thriving on his mother's milk. The stature of parents, while not wholly reliable, is the 'best' indication of the future size of the infant. Thus, if the infant does not appear to be gaining weight, but in all other respects seems to be happy and healthy, there should be no immediate cause for concern.

Other vital signs include:

1. Good skin colour; not grey or pale.
2. Alert and responsive.
3. Frequent 'wet' nappies with pale, odourless urine. (This sign is useful only if the baby is being exclusively breastfed, i.e. no supplementary or complementary feeds.)
4. Normal stools for age; see above.
5. Contented most of the time (i.e. not constantly fretful or crying) but without being lethargic.

Just as these can be considered positive signs in a baby who is not gaining weight, so too, if there is adequate weight gain but there are clear deficits in any of the above, there should be cause for concern.

References

Anand RK. The management of breastfeeding in a Bombay hospital. In: Assignment children 2, 55–56. Breastfeeding and Health. UNICEF; 1981:172.

Aono T, Aki T, Koike K, Kurachi K. Effects of sulpiride on poor lactation. Am J Obstet Gynecol 1982; 143:927–932.

Bass M, Kravath RE, Glass L. Death scene investigation in sudden infant death. N Engl J Med 1986; 315(2):100–105.

Bourne MA. Sleep and the newborn. New Generation 1983; 2(2):16–17.

Carvalho M et al. Effect of frequent breastfeeding on early milk production and infant weight gain. Pediatrics 1982; 72(3): 307–311.

Carvalho M et al. Does the duration and frequency of early breastfeeding affect nipple pain? Birth 1984; 11:2.

Clark G, Lincoln DW, Merrick L. Dopaminergic control of oxytocin release in lactating rats. J Endocrinol 1979; 83:409–420.

Coombe A. Management of infancy. New York: Fowlers and Wells; 1840:207. Cited in The Family Bed. Minneapolis: Thevenin.

Corsini GU. Evidence for dopamine receptors in the human brain mediating sedation and sleep. Life Sci 1977; 20(a):1613–1618.

Culley P, Milan P, Roginski C, Waterhouse J, Wood B. Are breast-fed babies still getting a raw deal in hospital? BMJ 1979; ii:891–893.

De Chateau P. The first hour after delivery. its impact on synchrony of parent-infant relationship. Pediatrician 1980; 9:151–168.

De Chateau P, Wiberg B. Long term effect on mother–infant behaviour of extra contact during the first hour post-partum. Acta Paediatr Scand 1977; 66:137–151.

Dewey KG, Lonnerdal B. Breast milk intake: variations in feeding practices. Am J Clin Nutr 1983; July:152–153 (letter).

Fisher C. In: Inch S, ed. Difficulties with breastfeeding – midwives in disarray? J R Soc Med 1987; 80:53–54.

Fleming PJ et al. Environment of infants during sleep and risk of sudden infant death syndrome:- results of 1993–1995 case–control study for Confidential Enquiry into Stillbirths and Deaths in Infancy. BMJ 1996; 313:191–195.

Foster K, Lader D, Cheesbrough S. Infant feeding 1995. Survey carried out for the Office of National Statistics. London: The Stationery Office; 1997.

Gardner D, Pearson J. A growth chart for premature and other infants. Arch Dis Child 1971; 46:783–787.

Garforth S, Garcia J. In: Inch S, ed. Difficulties with breastfeeding – midwives in disarray? J R Soc Med 1987; 80:53–57.

Glasier AS, McNeilly AS, Howie PW. The prolactin response to suckling. Clin Endocrinol 1984; 21:109–116.

Gunther M. Instinct and the nursing couple. Lancet 1955; i:575–578.

Hall B. Changing composition of milk and early development of an appetite control. Lancet 1975; i:779–781.

Howie PW. Breastfeeding – a new understanding. Midwives Chronicle and Nursing Notes 1985; July:184–192.

Hytten F. Clinical studies in lactation 11: variation in the major constituents during a feeding. BMJ 1954; i:176–179.

Illingworth RS, Stone DG. Self-demand feeding in a maternity unit. Lancet 1952; i:683–687.

Kauppila A, Kivinen S, Ylikorkala O. Metoclopramide increases prolactin release and milk secretion in the puerperium without stimulating the secretion of thyrotropin and thyroid hormones. J Clin Endocrinol Metab 1981; 52:436–439.

Kennedy KI. Consensus statement on the use of breastfeeding as a family planning method. Contraception 1989; 39:477.

King FT. Feeding and care of the baby. London: Macmillan; 1913.

Kries RV et al. Vitamin K content of maternal milk: influence of the stage of lactation, lipid composition and vitamin K supplements given to the mother. Pediatr Res 1987; 22(5).

Krnjevic K, Phillis JW. Pharmacological properties of ACh sensitive cells in the cerebral cortex. J Physiol 1963; 166:328–350.

Johnson NW. Breastfeeding at one hour of age. American Journal of Maternal and Child Nursing 1986; Jan/Feb:12–16.

Liddiard M. The mothercraft manual. London: J & A Churchill; 1924–1948.

Liedloff J. The continuum concept. London: Futura Publications; 1975.

Lucas A et al. Patterns of milk flow in breastfed babies. Lancet 1979; ii(8133): 57–58.

Macfarlane A. The psychology of childbirth. London: Fontana Open Books; 1977.

Martin J, Monk M. Infant feeding 1980. London: Office of Population Census and Surveys. Social Survey Division; 1982:40–44.

McNeilly AS, Robinson IC, Houston MJ, Howie PW. Release of prolactin and oxytocin in response to suckling. BMJ 1983; 287: 257–259.

Morley R, Abbott KA, Lucas A. Child Care Health Dev 1977; 23(6):475–478.

Naish L. Breastfeeding – its management and mismanagement. Lancet 1913; i:1657–1659.

Office of Population Censuses and Surveys. Mortality statistics by cause. Vol DH2. London: HMSO; 1985.

Olmsted RW, Jackson EB. Self-demand feeding in the first week of life. Pediatrics 1950; 6:396–401.

Paisley AC, Summerlee AJS. Relationships between behavioural states and activity in the cerebral cortex. Prog Neurobiol 1984; 22(2): 155–184.

Salariya EM, Robertson CM. The development of a neonatal stool colour comparator. Midwifery 1993; 9:35–40.

Salariya EM, Easton PM, Cater JI. Duration of feeding after early initiation and frequent feeding. Lancet 1978; ii:1141–1143.

Salver EJ. The effect of different feeding schedules on the growth of Bantu babies in the first week of life. J Trop Pediatr 1956; September: 97–102.

Simsarian FP, McLendon PA. Feeding behaviour of an infant during the first twelve weeks of life on a self-demand schedule. J Pediatr 1942; 20:93–103.

Simsarian FP, McLendon PA. Further records of the self-demand schedule in infant-feeding. J Pediatr 1945; 17:109–114.

Slaven S, Harvey D. Unlimited sucking time improves breastfeeding. Lancet 1981; i:392–393.

Thomsen ME, Hartstock TG, Larson C. The importance of immediate post-natal contact: its effects on breastfeeding. Can Fam Phys 1979; 25:1374–1378.

Urnas-Moberg K. The gastrointestinal tract in growth and reproduction. Sci Am 1989; July:60–65.

Weaver LT, Ewing G, Taylor LC. The bowel habits of milk fed infants. J Pediatr Gastroenterol Nutr 1988; 7:568–571.

White A, Freeth S, O'Brien M. Infant feeding 1990. Survey carried out for the DHSS by the Office of Population Censuses and Surveys. London: HMSO; 1992.

Whitehead RG, Paul AA. Growth charts and the assessment of infant feeding practices in the Western world and in developing countries. Early Hum Dev 1985; 9:187–207.

Whitfield MF, Kay R, Stevens S. Validity of routine clinical test weighing as a measure of the intake of breastfed infants. Arch Dis Child 1981; 56:919–921.

Widstrom AM, Ransjo-Arvidson AB, Christensson K et al. Gastric suction in healthy newborn infants. Acta Paediatr Scand 1987; 76:566–572.

Winters NW. The relationship of time of initial breastfeeding to success in breastfeeding. MA thesis, University of Washington; 1973.

Wood CS, Isaacs PC, Jensen M, Hilton HG. Exclusively breastfed infants: growth and calorie intake. Pediatr Nurs 1988; 14(2).

Woolridge M, Fisher C. Colic, 'overfeeding' and symptoms of lactose malabsorption in the breast-fed baby: a possible artefact of feed management? Lancet 1988; ii:382–384.

Woolridge MW et al. Individual patterns of milk intake during breast-feeding. Early Hum Dev 1982; 7:265–272.

Woolridge MW, Greasley V, Silpisornkosol S. The initiation of lactation: effect of early delayed contact for suckling on milk intake in the first week post-partum. A study in Chiang Mai, Northern Thailand. Early Hum Dev 1985; 12:269–278.

World Health Organization. An evaluation of infant growth: WHO Working Group on Infant Growth. (WHO/NUT/94.8). London: HMSO Publication Centre; 1994.

Ylikorkala O, Kauppila A, Kivinen S, Vinikka L. Sulpiride improves inadequate lactation. BMJ 1982; 285:249–250.

6 Factors that have been shown to be unhelpful

Additional fluids for breastfed babies   78
Test weighing   81
Unsubstantiated 'advice' to mothers in relation
    to food, drink and rest   82

Additional fluids for breastfed babies

Supplementary and complementary feeds of either water, glucose/dextrose or formula have not been shown in any of the trials reviewed below (or in any of the randomised controlled trials in the Cochrane Library of perinatal trials) to be of any benefit to healthy, term, breastfed infants.

Midwives should remember that bottle-feeding does not resolve breastfeeding problems, but that knowledgeable, enthusiastic and sympathetic help can.

Dehydration

The volume of colostrum/milk available to the newborn infant increases rapidly in the first 3 days after birth from a range of 7–122.5 mL per 24 h (Saint et al 1984) and a mean of 7.5 mL per feed in the first 24 h after birth, to a range of 98–775 mL per 24 h and a mean of 38 mL per feed by the third postnatal day (Houston et al 1983). There is no evidence to suggest that a healthy term baby has a need for large volumes of fluid any earlier than they are made available physiologically (Williams 1997).

To date, at least six trials have been undertaken to examine the suggestion that older healthy babies, who are exclusively breastfed, need extra water in hot weather. Studies measured the urine concentration of the babies, and found that it was well within the normal range and concluded that no additional water was necessary, even in hot weather (Almroth 1978, Almroth & Bidinger 1990, Armelini & Gonzales 1979, Ashraf et al 1993, Goldberg & Adams 1983, Sachdev et al 1991).

Jaundice

Various researchers have investigated the seemingly widespread belief that giving additional fluids to a breastfed baby prevents or resolves physiological jaundice. Nicoll et al (1982) randomly allocated 49 breastfed babies to three groups: no supplement, water supplement and dextrose supplement. Despite the observation that the infants in the dextrose group consumed a significantly greater mean volume of fluid than those in the water group, those in the no supplement group had the lowest mean serum bilirubin levels on the sixth day.

Carvalho et al (1981) compared two groups of breastfed babies, one of which received supplementary water and one of which did not, and Herrera (1984) similarly compared two groups, one of which received supplementary glucose while the other did not. They found no differences between the two groups in the number of babies that developed jaundice, the number that required phototherapy or in the mean serum bilirubin concentration.

Kuhr & Paneth (1982) recorded the total amount of supplementary dextrose given over a 72-h period to 77 consecutively born, healthy, term, breastfed babies, test weighed them on the fourth day and analysed the results in relation to those who appeared jaundiced and thus had their serum bilirubin levels measured. They found babies who took large volumes of dextrose supplement in the first 3 days of life not only tended to take less milk per feed by the fourth day, but were also more likely to be jaundiced than those who did not. None of the researchers found any relationship between the degree of weight loss and the development of physiological jaundice (Carvalho et al 1981, 1982, Herrera 1984, Kuhr & Paneth 1982).

On the basis of the evidence, the most effective way of reducing the incidence of physiological jaundice in breastfed babies would appear to be to ensure that no limitations are placed on the frequency with which the babies go to their mother's breast or on the duration of feeds.

Hypoglycaemia

Concern over the possibility that healthy term infants who feed infrequently in the first 24–48 h after birth might be at risk of developing hypoglycaemia has been addressed by UK national guidelines based on a World Health Organization-sponsored literature review (National Childbirth Trust 1997). These conclude that there is no evidence that long intervals between feeds adversely affects healthy term infants. Infants need not be screened for hypoglycaemia; neither do they need supplementary fluids.

Hazards of additional fluids

The fact that a practice cannot be shown to be of benefit ought to be sufficient reason for abandoning it, especially in the present economic climate. In 1980 it was estimated that a hospital that delivered 5000 babies per year, of whom 70% were initially breastfed, was paying out £7000 per year on prepacked supplementary feeds of water and dextrose (Kuhr & Paneth 1982).

More important still are the observations that supplementary fluids may ultimately reduce the length of time for which a mother breastfeeds her baby, either by undermining her confidence or by impairing her ability to establish effective lactation. The mechanism by which artificial feeding undermines the mother's attempts to breastfeed may be partly psychological, in that she becomes accustomed to seeing and measuring the quantity of milk taken by the baby. This, of course, is not necessary for successful breastfeeding, but the mother may doubt her ability to produce quantities of milk because she does not see it.

De Chateau et al (1977) compared two groups of breastfeeding women, one for whom test weighing and supplementation were routine, and one for whom this practice was discontinued. They found that five times as many mothers stopped breastfeeding in the first week in the supplemented group, and twice as many stopped in the second week. A year later, when the practice had been discontinued through the unit, they found that the mean duration of breastfeeding was 95 days, compared with the former 42 days.

Bergevin et al (1983) randomly allocated a large number of breastfeeding women into two groups: one group received a sample of formula when they left the hospital and the other did not. They found that even this small intervention was sufficient to increase the number of women who had stopped breastfeeding at 1 month, and who had introduced solids by 2 months. The difference between the two groups was even greater in 'vulnerable' groups, such as primiparae, the less well educated and those who became ill postnatally. Yet in many hospitals pre-packed feeds of even water and glucose bear the name of a manufacturer of infant formula, which in itself can act as a form of advertising (Lobstein 1987).

Both Herrera (1984) and Gray-Donald et al (1985) found significantly fewer women who were still breastfeeding at 4, 9 and 12 weeks after the birth of their babies, if their babies had received supplementary fluids in hospital, compared with those whose babies had been exclusively breastfed. This may, in turn, have repercussions on the future health of genetically susceptible infants (Borch-Johnsen et al 1984).

Although this remains controversial, the wishes of the parents should be respected. Many researchers have shown the value of exclusive breastfeeding to the children of parents with allergies (Evensen 1983, Minchin 1985, 1998, Jelliffe & Jelliffe 1978). Both cow's milk-based formula and soya-based formula are potential allergens, and even a single exposure may play a role in the aetiology of conditions such as eczema and 'wheezing'. Mothers should be advised not to use soya-based formula without seeking medical advice (Setchell et al 1997, UK Department of Health 1996).

Parents suffering from these conditions deserve every help in their attempts to avoid sensitising their children (Chandra et al 1986). If supplementation is essential for some reason, human milk will be less risky for such infants.

Test weighing

Under normal circumstances test weighing is neither a necessary nor an effective tool for assessing the adequacy of lactation. Test weighing is normally understood to mean calculating the amount of breast milk consumed at a feed by weighing the baby before and after that feed and subtracting the first weighing from the second.

Modern electronic scales are now available for weighing babies. The older type of mechanical scales have neither sufficient precision nor the accuracy necessary for measuring small intakes of breast milk. Their use can lead to errors of ± 30 g, which may be as large as the intake being measured (Culley et al 1979, Drewett et al 1984, Whitfield et al 1981).

It may also be positively harmful to a mother's confidence in her ability to breastfeed if a single test weighing appears to show that her baby has consumed what may be regarded as an inadequate volume. The measurement of only one feed may be unrepresentative of other feeds taken throughout the day (Houston et al 1983).

Measuring only volume intake, without a knowledge of the calorie content of the milk consumed, may give a misleading picture of the nutritional adequacy of the baby's diet.

If it is necessary to know how much milk a breastfed baby is consuming, test weighing should be carried out over a complete 24-h period, using an electronic, averaging scale (or a heavily 'damped' electronic scale) in order to establish the volume intake accurately.

Unsubstantiated 'advice' to mothers in relation to food, drink and rest

The advice given to breastfeeding women concerning their optimum food and drink intake has long been the subject of debate, and in this area, as in so many others, much of the advice has been conflicting.

Additional fluids for breastfeeding mothers

In the 1950s researchers demonstrated that a baby's weight was not significantly improved by deliberately increasing the mother's fluid intake (Illingworth & Kilpatrick 1953). More recently, other studies have shown that neither a significant decrease (Dearlove & Dearlove 1981) nor a significant increase (Dearlove & Dearlove 1981, Dusdieker et al 1985, Morse et al 1992) in maternal fluid intake has any effect on milk production.

Thirst effectively regulates the fluid intake of a lactating woman, just as it does with all other lactating mammals, and the practice of encouraging breastfeeding women to drink large quantities of liquid should be abandoned. They might, however, be reminded that dark, strongly smelling urine is an indication that they need to drink more.

Additional calories for breastfeeding mothers

It has become apparent over the past few years that the theoretical calculation of the number of extra calories that a lactating woman needs to obtain from her diet is not borne out in practice. This calculation was based on an assumption that to provide 800 mL of milk (560 calories) she would have to make some 700 calories available for milk production (the efficiency of milk production being about 80%) (National Research Council 1980)

Recent dietary surveys in developed countries performed on well-nourished women with healthy babies have consistently found their calorie intake to be less than the recommended amount (Butte et al 1984, Whitehead et al 1981). Furthermore, controlled trials conducted in developing countries have demonstrated that giving extra food to mothers, even those who were poorly nourished, did not increase the rate of growth of their babies (Blackwell et al 1973, Delgado et al 1982, Prentice et al 1980, 1983a,b).

A possible explanation for these findings has been supplied by Illingworth et al (1986), who found that metabolic efficiency was enhanced in lactating women, who were therefore able to conserve energy and 'subsidise' the cost of their milk production.

Mothers who wish to undertake strenuous exercise (from 6–8 weeks after birth) can be reassured that this will have no effect on either the volume or composition of their milk (Dewey et al 1994).

Hunger will effectively regulate the calorie intake of a breastfeeding woman, just as it does in all other lactating mammals, and the practice of encouraging breastfeeding mothers to eat excessively should be abandoned. They might, however, need advice regarding the nature of a 'well-balanced diet', which is so often recommended without further explanation.

If healthy breastfeeding women wish to lose weight, they can be reassured that a modest weight loss (1–2 lbs per week) will not affect lactation (Dusdieker et al 1994, Strode et al

1986). Exclusive breastfeeding combined with a low-fat diet and exercise will result in more effective weight loss than diet and exercise alone (Dewey 1998, Hammer et al 1996).

It is worth noting that a poor appetite postnatally can be an indication of specific clinical states. As milk production would appear to 'drive' appetite, rather than the reverse, poor appetite may indicate poor milk production. Poor appetite may also be associated with postnatal depression and with clinical states such as thyroid or pituitary dysfunction.

Dietary prohibitions for breastfeeding mothers

As a general rule, there is no reason to advise a lactating woman that she should omit any particular food from her diet, just because she is breastfeeding. Any food may be consumed in moderation, unless or until the situation dictates otherwise. However, a woman with a family history of allergy or intolerance may benefit from some modification of her diet, during both pregnancy and lactation (Chandra et al 1986).

She should be reassured that the very loose stools that her baby may have from the third to the fifth day of life are a perfectly normal response to the influx of milk that occurs at this time, and are unlikely to be related to maternal dietary indiscretions.

However, it appears that some foods may have an allergenic effect on particular babies when ingested by their mothers (Chandra et al 1986, Gerrard 1980). If there is any reason to suspect that any food the mother has eaten has been responsible for some adverse reaction in the baby, she should avoid that food for 2 weeks and then return to it. If the baby's condition deteriorates again, the mother should avoid the food completely and seek additional dietary advice (Cant et al 1986).

References

Almroth SG. Water requirements of breastfed babies in a hot climate. Am J Clin Nutr 1978; 31:1154–1157.

Almroth S, Bidinger PD. No need for water supplementation for exclusively breastfed infants under hot and arid conditions. Trans R Soc Trop Med Hyg 1990; 84:602–604.

Armelini PA, Gonzales CF. Breastfeeding and fluid intake in a hot climate. Clin Pediatr 1979; 18:425–426.

Ashraf RN et al. Additional water is not needed for healthy breastfed babies in a hot climate. Acta Paediatr Scand 1993; 82: 1007–1011.

Bergevin Y, Dougherty C, Kramer MS. Do infant formula samples shorten the duration of breastfeeding? Lancet 1983; i: 1148–1151.

Blackwell RQ, Chow BF, Chinn KSK, Blackwell BN. Prospective maternal nutrition study in Taiwan: rationale, study design feasibility and preliminary findings. Nutr Rep Int 1973; 7: 517–532.

Borch-Johnsen K et al. Relation between breastfeeding and incidence rates of insulin dependent diabetes mellitus. Lancet 1984; ii:1083–1086.

Butte NF, Garza C, Stuff JE, Smith EO, Bichos BJ. Effect of maternal diet and body composition on lactational performance. Am J Clin Nutr 1984; 39:296–306.

Cant AJ, Bailes JA, Marsden RA, Hewitt D. Effect of maternal dietary exclusion on breastfed infants with eczema: two controlled studies. BMJ 1986; 293:231–233.

Carvalho M et al. Effect of water supplementation on physiological jaundice in breastfed babies. Arch Dis Child 1981; 56(7):568–569.

Carvalho M et al. Frequency of breastfeeding and serum bilirubin concentration. Am J Dis Child 1982; 136:737–738.

Chandra RK, Puri S, Suraika C et al. Influence of maternal food avoidance during pregnancy and lactation on the incidence of atopic eczema in infants. Clin Allergy 1986; 16:563–569.

Culley P, Milan P, Roginski C, Waterhouse J, Wood B. Are breastfed babies still getting a raw deal in hospital? BMJ 1979; 2:891–893.

De Chateau P et al. A study of factors promoting and inhibiting lactation. Dev Med Child Neurol 1977; 19:575–584.

Dearlove JC, Dearlove BM. Prolactin, fluid balance and lactation. Br J Obstet Gynaecol 1981; 123:845–846.

Delgado HL, Marmtorell R, Klein RE. Nutrition, lactation and birth interval components in rural Guatemala. Am J Clin Nutr 1982; 35:1468–1476.

Dewey KG. Effects of maternal caloric retriction and exercise during lactation. J Nutr 1998; 128(2 Suppl):386S–389S.

Dewey KG, Lovelady CA, Nommsen-Rivers LA et al. A randomised study of the effects of aerobic exercise by lactating women on breast-milk volume and composition. N Engl J Med 1994; 330(7):449–453.

Drewett RF, Woolridge MW, Greasley V et al. Evaluating breast-milk intake by test weighing: a portable electronic balance suitable for community and field studies. Early Hum Dev 1984; 10:123–126.

Dusdieker LB et al. Effect of supplementary fluids on human milk production. J Pediatr 1985; 106:207–211.

Dusdieker LB, Hemingway DL, Stumbo PJ. Is milk production impaired by dieting during lactation? Am J Clin Nutr 1994; 59: 833–840.

Evensen S. Relationship between infant morbidity and breastfeeding versus artificial feeding in industrialized countries: a review of the literature. World Health Organization Regional Office for Europe. ICP NUT 010/6 Rev. 1 0292M; 1983 (obtainable by mail order from HMSO Publications Centre, 51 Nine Elms Lane, London SW8 5DR, UK).

Gerrard JW. Adverse reactions to foods in breastfed babies. In: Freier S, Eidelman A, eds. Human milk – its biological and social value. Selected papers from the International Symposium on Breastfeeding, Tel Aviv; 1980:170–175.

Goldberg NM, Adams E. Supplementary water for breastfed babies in a hot dry climate – not really a necessity. Arch Dis Child 1983; January:73–74.

Gray-Donald K et al. Effect of formula supplementation in hospital on the duration of breastfeeding: a controlled trial. Pediatrics 1985; 75(3):514–518.

Hammer RL, Babcock G, Fisher AG. Low-fat diet and exercise in obese lactating women. Breastfeeding Rev 1996; 4(1):29–34.

Herrera AJ. Supplemented versus unsupplemented breastfeeding. Perinatology – Neonatology 1984; 8(3):70–71.

Houston MJ et al. Factors affecting the duration of breastfeeding: 1. Measurement of breast milk intake in the first week of life. Early Hum Dev 1983; 8:49–54.

Illingworth PJ, Jong RT, Howie PW, Leslie P, Isles TE. Diminution in energy expenditure during lactation. BMJ 1986; 292: 437–441.

Illingworth RS, Kilpatrick B. Lactation and fluid intake. Lancet 1953; ii:1175–1177.

Jelliffe DD, Jelliffe EFP. Human milk in the modern world. London: Oxford University Press; 1978.

Kuhr M, Paneth N. Feeding practices and early neonatal jaundice. J Pediatr Gastroenterol Nutr 1982; 1:485–488.

Lobstein T. Warding off the bottle. London: London Food Commission; 1987.

Minchin M. Food for thought – a parent's guide to food intolerance. Oxford: Oxford University Press; 1985.

Minchin M. Breastfeeding matters: what we need to know about infant feeding. Melbourne: Alma Publications; 1998.

Morse JM, Ewing G, Gamble D, Donahue P. The effect of maternal fluid intake on breast milk supply: a pilot study. Can J Public Health 1992; 83(3):213–216.

National Childbirth Trust. Hypoglycaemia of the newborn. Guidelines for appropriate blood glucose screening of breast and bottle fed babies in the United Kingdom. London: National Childbirth Trust; 1997.

National Research Council. Recommended dietary allowances. 9th edn. Washington: National Academy of Sciences; 1980.

Nicoll A et al. Supplementary feeding and jaundice in newborns. Acta Paediatr Scand 1982; 71:759–761.

Olsen A. Nursing under conditions of thirst or excessive ingestion of fluid. Acta Obstet Gynecol Scand 1940; 20:313–343.

Prentice AM, Roberts SB, Whitehead RG. Dietary supplementation of Gambian nursing mothers and lactational performance. Lancet 1980; ii:886–888.

Prentice AM, Whitehead RG, Roberts SB. Dietary supplementation of lactating Gambian women. i. Effect on breastmilk volume and quality. Hum Nutr Clin Nutr 1983a; 37(c):53–64.

Prentice AM, Lunn PG, Watkinson M, Whitehead RG. Dietary supplementation of lactating Gambian women. ii. Effect on maternal health, nutritional status and biochemistry. Hum Nutr Clin Nutr 1983b; 37(c):65–74.

Sachdev HPS et al. Water supplementation in exclusively breastfed infants during summer in the tropics. Lancet 1991; 337: 929–933.

Saint L et al. The yield and nutrient content of colostrum and milk of women from giving birth to one month post partum. Br J Nutr 1984; 52:87–95.

Setchell KDR, Zimmer-Nechemias L, Cai J, Heubi JE. Exposure of infants to phyto-oestrogens from soy-based infant formula. Lancet 1997; 350:23–27.

Strode MA, Dewey KG, Lonnerdal B. Effects of short term caloric restriction on lactational performance of well nourished mothers. Acta Paediatr Scand 1986; 75(2):222–229.

UK Department of Health. Advice on soy-based infant formula. DH 96/244. London: HMSO; 1996.

Whitehead RG, Paul AA, Black AE, Wiles SJ. Recommended dietary amounts of energy for pregnancy or lactation in the UK. In: Torun B, Young VR, Rang WM, eds. Protein energy requirements of developing countries: evaluation of new data. Tokyo: United Nations University; 1981:259–265.

Whitfield MF, Kay R, Stevens S. Validity of routine test weighing as a measure of the intake of breastfed infants. Arch Dis Child 1981; 56:919–921.

Williams AF. Hypoglycaemia of the newborn – review of the literature. Geneva: Division of Child Health and Development, and Maternal and Newborn Health/Safe Motherhood, World Health Organization; 1997.

Protecting breastfeeding 7

Provision of free samples to mothers   89
Promotion of breastmilk substitutes   90
Baby-Friendly Hospital initiative and the Ten Steps   92

Provision of free samples to mothers

Giving infant formula to breastfed babies in their first week of life has been found to be the most important variable predicting the cessation of breastfeeding in the first 2 weeks (White et al 1992). It has also been shown that giving samples of formula to breastfeeding mothers is likely to shorten the period for which they breastfeed, as well as encouraging the early introduction of solid food (Bergevin et al 1983). Lactational failure in this context is a result of the combined effects of lack of confidence and reduced suckling (Houston & Howie 1981).

Giving free samples to mothers can also imply recommendation of a brand, and thus becomes an effective way of promoting brand sales (Hamilton & Whinnett 1986). It also raises doubts in the mother's mind about the degree to which those caring for her are committed to breastfeeding. There is no reason why breastfeeding mothers of healthy term infants should be given samples of ready-to-feed formula, water or glucose, even in hospital. They should not be given to any mother on discharge from hospital and particularly not to breastfeeding mothers.

In the UK, women who wish to bottle-feed and who are receiving Income Support are entitled to milk tokens under the Welfare Food Scheme, which can be exchanged for 900 g of infant formula per week. This should be adequate for any baby who is bottle-fed, and it should not be necessary for the mother to be given free samples by the hospital when she goes home.

Women who are receiving Working Families' Tax Credit can buy infant formula at a reduced rate at clinics and approved pharmacies.

Promotion of breastmilk substitutes

WHO code

As a result of international collaboration between the World Health Organization (WHO), the United Nations International Children's Emergency Fund (UNICEF), medical experts, government representatives, infant food industry personnel and the consumer groups, a voluntary Code for the Marketing of Breastmilk Substitutes was developed (WHO 1981). The Code seeks to contribute to safe, adequate nutrition for infants, to promote and protect breastfeeding, to ensure the correct use of breastmilk substitutes and to control the use of questionable marketing techniques in the selling of products for bottle-feeding.

The Code does not prevent mothers from bottle-feeding if that is what they choose to do. The object of the Code is to control unethical marketing to parents and staff in healthcare facilities, and to reduce the pressure that some companies exert on health professionals. It seeks to encourage and maintain the woman's right to breastfeed, and the baby's right to have access to its mother's own milk. Nowhere does it seek to enforce breastfeeding. The Code applies to all breastmilk substitutes for babies, including follow-on milks and other products that can be given in a feeding bottle, as well as utensils used for bottle-feeding, such as feeding bottles and teats.

Included in the Articles of the Code are:

1. No advertising of these products to the public.
2. No free samples to mothers or members of their families.
3. No promotion of products in healthcare facilities.
4. No company personnel to advise mothers or members of their families.
5. No gifts or personal samples to health workers.
6. No words or pictures idealising bottle-feeding, including pictures of infants on the labels of the products.
7. All information on infant feeding, including product labels,

should explain the benefits of breastfeeding and the costs and hazards associated with bottle-feeding.

8. Unsuitable products, such as sweetened condensed milk, should not be promoted for babies.
9. All products should be of high quality and should take into account the climatic and storage conditions of the country where they are to be used.

The Code recommends that healthcare facilities and staff should not be used for the purposes of advertising and promoting bottle-feeding to the public. This recommendation includes the display of calendars and posters, as well as the use of cot tags, tape measures, leaflets, baby booklets and mugs.

At the 1981 World Health Assembly, Britain voted in favour of the WHO Code. It is an international code and therefore applies worldwide. It was set down as a minimum requirement to protect infant health, and it is the responsibility of national governments to formulate their Codes based on the WHO Code.

On 1 March 1995 the Infant Formula and Follow-on Formula Regulations 1995, Statutory Instruments 1995 No. 77, came into force. This law includes regulations regarding advertising. It forbids the use of pictures of infants in the labelling of infant formulae or other pictures or text that may idealise the use of the product. It allows the advertising of infant formulae in publications specialising in baby care and distributed through the healthcare system, in scientific publications and for the purposes of trade before the retail stage.

Such materials must include clear information about:

- the benefits and superiority of breastfeeding
- the possible negative effect on breastfeeding of introducing partial bottle-feeding
- the difficulty of reversing the decision not to breastfeed.

During the consultation stages, 48 agencies, including the British Medical Association, the Royal College of Midwives and the British Paediatric Association, supported the proposal that there should be a total ban of advertising baby milks. Their efforts were unsuccessful, although the advertising of infant formulae is not allowed in premises where it is sold, nor can free samples be given.

It is easy to understand why mothers may gain the impression that bottle-feeding is equivalent to breastfeeding if the health-care facility endorses such practices.

Baby-Friendly Hospital initiative and the Ten Steps

Breastfeeding practices are currently being rigorously reassessed by hospitals that want to achieve the prestigious UNICEF UK Baby-Friendly Hospital Award. This requires (and independently verifies) that the hospital fully implements the 'Ten Steps to Successful Breastfeeding' (see Appendix 1). Baby-Friendly Hospitals are also required to implement the International (WHO) Code on the Marketing of Breastmilk Substitutes.

References

Bergevin Y, Dougherty C, Kramer MS. Do infant formula samples shorten breastfeeding? Lancet 1983; i:1148–1151.

Hamilton R, Whinnett D. A comparison of the WHO and United Kingdom Codes of Practice for Marketing of Breastmilk Substitutes. Lancaster: University of Lancaster; 1986.

Houston MJ, Howie PW. The importance of support for the breast-feeding mother. Health Visitor 1981; 54(6):243.

White A, Freeth S, O'Brien M. Infant feeding 1990. London: Office of Population Censuses and Surveys, Social Survey Division; 1992.

World Health Organization. International Code of Marketing of Breastmilk Substitutes. Geneva: WHO; 1981.

Antenatal and postnatal considerations

Influencing the decision to breastfeed	93
Sustaining the decision to breastfeed	95
Prevention of feeding problems	96
Postnatal care of the breasts	98
Treatment of sore nipples	99
Hand expression	102
Prevention and treatment of engorgement	103
Prevention and treatment of mastitis	105

Influencing the decision to breastfeed

In this society, the majority of women who decide to breastfeed seem to make this decision before they are pregnant or very early in pregnancy (Beske & Garvis 1982, Goodine & Fried 1984, Ladas 1970, Mackey & Fried 1981). Those who choose to bottle-feed tend to make up their minds later in pregnancy (Beske & Garvis 1982).

Giving well-designed, written and illustrated information about breastfeeding to women has been shown to increase (or reinforce) their knowledge of the subject, but it is unlikely to affect their choice of feeding method, or to increase the duration of breast-feeding (Kaplowitz 1983). It is more likely that their choice will be affected by socially acquired attitudes and the support that they feel they will get from their families and friends (Hoddinott & Pill 1999, Ladas 1970, Littman et al 1994, Switzky et al 1979). Persuasive campaigns in the mass media and in clinics have been found to have little effect on feeding practices (Gueri et al 1979, Kirk 1979, Svejcar 1977). Furthermore, once a woman has decided how she will feed her baby, she is unlikely to change her mind (Kaplowitz 1983), although the impact of information indicating that bottle-feeding is problematic has not yet been tested.

As can be seen from pages 96–98, no form of antenatal preparation of the breasts has been shown to be of benefit; thus, asking a woman in early pregnancy how she plans to feed her baby is not only unnecessary, it may even be counterproductive if she has not already decided to breastfeed and feels pressured into making a decision. Furthermore, the question 'Are you going to breast or bottle feed?' implies that the two methods are equivalent.

If, in the course of the discussion between mother and midwife, it becomes apparent that the mother would like more information, then this should be provided; otherwise, it could be safely left until the last trimester of pregnancy.

Midwives who feel strongly that 'breast is best' have a difficult task in giving information to women who are undecided about their feeding method, or who have chosen to bottle-feed. At no stage should the mother be given the impression that bottle-feeding is equivalent to breastfeeding, or that it is without risk.

In particular, women with a strong family history of allergy should be informed that their decision to breastfeed may prevent serious illness in their children. However, there is a subtle but important difference between the heavy-handed approach that makes mothers feel guilty, and the more sensitive approach that allows mothers to make their own decision. The Informed Choice leaflet 'Feeding your baby: breast or bottle?' may be helpful in this regard (Midwives Information and Resource Service/NHS Centre 1999).

Antenatal classes

One study has demonstrated that one antenatal breastfeeding class, given in the last 2 months of pregnancy to women who have already decided to breastfeed, had a significant positive effect, not only on the duration of breastfeeding but on the way in which the mother perceived herself and her baby postnatally (Wiles 1984). This class (given by an enthusiastic midwife) contained information on the anatomy and physiology of lactation (see pp. 28–32), how to breastfeed (see pp. 43–51), self-care of the breastfeeding mother, possible setbacks early in breastfeeding and their treatments (see pp. 101–112), breastfeeding and the working mother, and resources for the breastfeeding mother (how to get help from both professional and voluntary organisations).

This finding has recently been replicated by Duffy et al (1997) and by the CRIB project (Shanahan 2001 – personal communication), a study funded by the Department of Health as part of the Infant Feeding Initiative.

Sustaining the decision to breastfeed

In addition to factors already mentioned, such as early contact and early suckling, other aspects of postnatal care have also been shown to increase the length of time for which a woman breast-feeds. In one study a group of women who were given a short, personal, bedside teaching session while still in hospital were compared with two others: one group just received a card with the name and phone number of a professional feeding adviser, and women in the other group were given the same card plus a manual containing the sort of information that had been given at the teaching session.

Significantly more women who had received the individual tuition were still breastfeeding at 1 month postpartum, compared with the other two groups (Johnson et al 1984). The effectiveness of this personal, professional contact should encourage midwives to give this aspect of their role high priority.

Other studies have identified the baby and the baby's father as the greatest sources of encouragement to the mother's breast-feeding attempts (Beske & Garvis 1982, Littman et al 1994), and the woman's own mother as the greatest source of discouragement if she herself had not breastfed (Beske & Garvis 1982). The findings of both of these studies could be utilised if the personal, professional helping session were given at the first feed, in the peace and quiet after the newly delivered mother and baby had been attended to and made clean and comfortable, and while the father was still present.

The baby's behaviour and needs can be explained to the usually highly receptive parents, so that in future the baby will not be regarded as being in any way critical or manipulative. The mother's breast and nipple can be considered in relation to the baby's mouth, head and body; the importance of correct positioning and the concept of supply and demand briefly explained (Houston 1985). (For further details of the first teaching session, see pp. 53–58.)

The other factor that has been shown to be of benefit is prolonged, intermittent, postnatal contact with the mother (Sjolin et al 1979). Despite the fact that the study in question was not designed to promote breastfeeding by means of this intervention, but to discover why women stopped breastfeeding, the researchers found that more women in the group who were telephoned weekly (in order to be interviewed) throughout the period of breastfeeding were still breastfeeding at 6 months, compared with a control group who were interviewed retrospectively. If the interviewer discovered that the woman being telephoned had a problem, it was possible to offer immediate, competent, practical help. This is a role that the voluntary breastfeeding organisations could effectively undertake (perhaps in some modified form), if contact could be made with the mother in the early postnatal period. One of the advantages of extending midwifery care to 28 days is that the mother receives prolonged, intermittent contact, as well as more consistent advice. With good interprofessional communication, these advantages should continue when the care of the mother and baby passes to the health visitor.

Prevention of feeding problems

Breastfeeding is a normal physiological process – a natural consequence of giving birth – and in many countries is still the only reliable means of ensuring the survival and healthy growth of a newborn baby.

Breastfeeding problems are likely only when the physiological process is impeded, either by surrounding it with rules and regulations, or by failing to attach the baby to the breast correctly (see pp. 49–51). However, where this has not been understood, an explanation that is frequently given for the prevalence of breastfeeding problems in Western cultures – despite the lack of evidence to support it – is that they are due to the thinness or sensitivity of the nipple skin. This misconception has unfortunately formed the basis of most of the advice given, and breast preparation advocated, in the antenatal and postnatal period.

Antenatal preparation

Nipple soreness is not related to the mother's colouring, nor to the toughness of her skin. There is no evidence to support the commonly held belief that fair-skinned women are more likely to experience nipple problems (Brockway 1986, Gans 1958, Brown & Hurlock 1975). The persistence of this myth may result in unjustifiable numbers of fair-, red- and auburn-haired women being dissuaded from breastfeeding, and problems (should they occur in such women) being regarded as unavoidable.

Nipple shape

Although antenatal examination of the breasts may have some predictive value, many women with poorly protractile nipples will be able to breastfeed successfully without treatment (Hytten 1954). They will probably need particular help with attaching their baby to the breast during the first feeds.

As the nipple plays little active part in the mechanism of milk release (see p. 30–31), breastfeeding success is likely to have more to do with good attachment than with nipple shape.

Nipple preparation

Although there are many variations in the recommended practices, they all fall into three major categories: some form of nipple friction, application of various creams or antenatal expression of colostrum. These practices have been evaluated by a number of researchers (Clark 1985, L'Esperance 1980, Brown & Hurlock 1975, Whitley 1978), and no evidence has been found to support any of them.

The arguments on which they are based have been further undermined by studies that have found no differences between the incidence of nipple problems between multiparous and primiparous women (Gunther 1945, Jones 1984, Nicholson 1985), which would be expected if nipple 'toughening' were effective.

Nipple preparation for inverted and non-protractile nipples

Attempts to improve nipple protractility by the use of shells or stretching 'exercises' have been shown to be of no value (Alexander et al 1992, MAIN Trial Collaborative Group 1994). Furthermore, 45% of the women recruited to the control groups in the MAIN trial, and who therefore did nothing to their inverted or flat nipples in pregnancy, were still breastfeeding at 6 weeks postpartum, which compares favourably with 39% in the general population (White et al 1992). See also the section on inverted nipples in Chapter 9.

Expression of colostrum

There is no justification for advising pregnant women to express colostrum regularly, on the grounds that it will improve subsequent lactation. Not only does it have no effect on milk flow or milk production (Beske & Garvis 1982, Ingelman-Sundberg 1958, Waller et al 1941) but it may dispose women to mastitis if the breast is traumatised (Ingelman-Sundberg 1958). On the other hand, there is no reason why a woman who wishes to satisfy her curiosity as to the nature of colostrum should be dissuaded from doing so (gently).

A pregnant woman who intends to breastfeed should be advised that no physical preparation of her breasts can ensure trouble-free feeding. Instead she should be taught the principles of good breastfeeding technique, and to regard any pain she may experience not as inevitable, but as a signal that she needs to improve her technique.

Postnatal care of the breasts

Cleanliness

Washing the breasts before each feed is no longer recommended, and mothers should be advised that adequate personal hygiene is all that is necessary. The use of soap, and the use of alcohol, have both been shown to increase the incidence of nipple soreness (Newton 1952). Sprays containing alcohol and chlorhexidine are ineffective in preventing nipple trauma (Herd & Feeney 1986, Inch & Fisher 1987, Slaven et al 1987).

Creams and ointments

Of those that have been tested in controlled trials, stilboestrol cream and vitamin A and D concentrate (cod liver oil) have been shown to increase the incidence of nipple damage (Gans 1958, Newton 1952); lanolin, vitamin A and D ointment, vitamin B ointment (both in lanolin and petroleum base) and water-repellent silicone barrier cream have been shown to be ineffective in preventing nipple damage (Gans 1958, Newton 1952, Shurtz et al 1978). Tincture of benzoin, although not formally tested, contains 75–80% alcohol and might therefore be expected to increase the incidence of nipple damage. It is likely that any cream will alter the skin ecology in some way (Minchin 1985), and its use must always be justified.

As there seems to be little evidence that any of the creams, ointments, sprays or tinctures frequently advocated is of any value in preventing nipple soreness, attention should be paid to ensuring that the baby is correctly attached during breastfeeding.

Limiting sucking time

This practice, which was first advocated in the early 1900s, was also a product of the mistaken belief that nipples needed toughening to promote pain-free feeding. Recent studies have shown that nipple soreness is not affected by the duration of the feed, but that limiting sucking time is likely to have an adverse effect on breastfeeding as a whole (Carvalho et al 1984, Slaven & Harvey 1981).

Treatment of sore nipples

A study of practice in the early 1980s found that most methods of treatment advocated at that time (Garcia & Garforth 1985) fell into two groups: (1) those that aimed to heal the nipple by putting something on it (the 'magic wand' treatments), and (2) those that aimed to allow the nipple to heal spontaneously by removing or reducing the cause of the damage. No randomised controlled trial (RCT) has yet been done to assess the usefulness of any of the creams, sprays, lotions or ointments that, according to Garcia & Garforth's study (1985), were often recommended by midwives as treatments for sore nipples; there is thus no scientific basis for their use. Nor is there any scientific evidence to support the use of expressed breast milk or colostrum on the nipples after feeding (Hewat & Ellis 1987, Pugh et al 1996).

Only one RCT was identified which assessed the effectiveness of methods designed to remove or reduce damage (Nicholson 1985) and this compared three methods: (1) taking the baby off the breast and expressing the milk, (2) the use of a nipple shield, and (3) repositioning the baby at the breast (although precisely what was understood by this term was not clearly defined).

Over the 48–h period of the trial all methods were equally acceptable in producing nipple healing, but the use of the nipple shield proved to be highly unacceptable to mothers. Additionally, the use of a thick red rubber nipple shield had also been shown to reduce significantly the amount of milk available to the baby (Woolridge et al 1980). There can be even less justification for the use of bottle teats as nipple shields, as they are likely further to reduce physiological milk removal and maternal breast stimulation.

Resting, expressing and repositioning (reattachment)

The two methods that did seem acceptable to the majority of mothers allocated to each one – 'repositioning' and 'resting and expressing' – were equally effective in producing nipple healing over the 48 h of the trial. Thus, with both treatments, the nipple had ceased to be traumatised.

However, the long-term objective of treating sore nipples is to facilitate pain-free, successful breastfeeding. Logically, removing the baby from the breast will heal sore nipples, but only in the same way that not breastfeeding at all will 'prevent' them. Furthermore, removing the baby from the breast in order to heal nipples creates the immediate problem of maintaining milk production. A breast pump applies negative pressure to the end of the nipple, but it does not directly stimulate the nerve endings in the breast. Thus the prolactin surge that normally follows suckling (and is responsible, in part, for milk synthesis) is reduced when a breast pump is used (Howie et al 1980, Zinaman et al 1992). See also Chapter 10 'Establishing lactation with an electric pump'.

The other components in the maintenance of lactation are the effective removal of milk in response to the milking action provided by the baby's tongue and jaw (absent if a pump is used) and the active expulsion of milk in response to oxytocin release – the 'let-down' reflex.

Less milk will be obtained from the breast in response to periodic expression compared with direct suckling (Freidman & Sachtleben 1961). (This deficit was reduced in the past by giving nasal oxytocin to mothers who needed to use a breast pump for any length of time (Ruis 1981), but this treatment is no longer available in the UK.) On both counts, therefore, milk production begins to decline. (The use of a breast pump should not be assumed to be a totally atraumatic process; in the trial referred to above (Nicholson 1985), four of the six women with new nipple cracks at the end of 48 h had been using a breast pump.)

Thus, in terms of achieving the long-term goal of pain-free, successful lactation, paying close attention to feeding technique ('repositioning') is likely to be far more effective than removing the baby from the breast ('resting and expressing').

Damaged nipples and moist wound healing

The frequently repeated advice to expose nipples to the air to aid healing is not supported by research. There is evidence that a superficial, clean wound will heal more rapidly if it is kept moist (Winter & Scales 1963). This is now the basis of modern wound healing (Alper et al 1983, Anonymous 1988). Small amounts of lanolin (purified to reduce the risk of adverse skin reactions) or soft white paraffin (either as an ointment or as squares of sterilised paraffin-impregnated gauze) applied to the nipple (and covered with a breast pad) prevent the damaged area from drying out. The cause of the damage must be treated concurrently if the nipples are to heal.

If the damaged area has become superficially infected, paraffin gauze (also impregnated with fucidic acid) may be useful.

Although there is a strong theoretical basis for these treatments, they have yet to be evaluated in the context of RCTs. There is no evidence to support the use of any creams, sprays or ointments, antenatally or postnatally, to prevent or treat nipple soreness (see p. 100).

Nipple shields

Nipple shields should not be used as a substitute for teaching the mother how to correct the problem of sore nipples by improving her feeding technique. Their use in the early days of lactation may lead to a conditioned rejection of the breast by the baby, which can be extremely difficult to correct. Prolonged use may also adversely affect the mother's milk supply, as less milk is made available to the baby as a result of less efficient milking action of the baby's tongue and jaw through the flange of the shield. This was particularly true of the traditional thick rubber nipple shields (Woolridge et al 1980). (As yet there is no evidence on which to base statements about the effectiveness of silicone shields.)

Clinical experience suggests that some mothers may benefit from the judicious use of a thin silicone shield, principally if their nipples have been severely traumatised by incorrect attachment, and they choose not to 'rest and express'. They should bear in mind that milk transfer may be impaired (Woolridge et al 1980), so that the baby may need to feed for longer and/or more often. Nipple shields should never be used before the milk has 'come in', 2–5 days after delivery.

Hand expression

All breastfeeding women should be offered the opportunity to learn how to hand express. This will be of value to them if they are concerned that their child has not fed as often as they would like in the first 24–48 h and wish to express colostrum. It will also be a useful alternative to a breast pump if they wish to express milk for any reason, for example if the breasts are so full that it is difficult to attach the baby, or if they wish to leave some milk for their baby to be fed in their absence.

How to help a mother to hand express

1. Suggest that she sits comfortably, with her back straight.
2. Suggest that she places her little finger at the base of her breast, against her ribs, and spreads her other fingers slightly to support her breast. Her thumb will be on top.
3. Suggest that she adjusts her fingers, if necessary, to ensure that her first finger and thumb are opposite each other, making a big 'C' shape around her breast.
4. Remind her that the milk comes from deep within the breast, so her finger and thumb need to be well away from the nipple.
5. Tell her to squeeze her thumb and first finger gently together, hold the squeeze for a count of 3, and release, but not to change the position of her finger and thumb.
6. Encourage her to repeat the squeezing and releasing until she sees drops of colostrum/milk appearing at the nipple. Tell her to be patient as it may take a minute or two for her efforts to be rewarded.
7. Some women find hand expressing more effective if they press their whole hand back and in towards the breast just before they squeeze.

8. She should avoid sliding her thumb over the skin of her breast, as too vigorous an action may damage the skin.
9. If her fingers get tired, suggest that she changes hands, or changes breasts.
10. If the milk flow slows, suggest that she rotates her hand slightly and tries a different section of the breast before changing breasts.
11. Collect the milk in a sterile, wide-mouthed container.

It is easier for the woman to learn how to express if someone guides her rather than just gives her a sheet of instructions (Fig. 8.1).

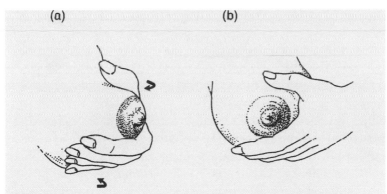

Figure 8.1 How to hand express. Reproduced by permission of the Women's Centre, Oxford

Prevention and treatment of engorgement

The term engorgement needs to be defined because different people mean different things by it.

Vascular engorgement

Because lactation is anticipated, the body prepares the breast anatomically and physiologically (Smith 1974). During the course of pregnancy, ductal and alveolar growth is stimulated (and milk secretion inhibited) by the high levels of placental oestrogen in the mother's bloodstream. When, after placental delivery, this has fallen to a point where it can no longer inhibit the action of prolactin, synthesis and secretion of milk can begin. This requires extensive cardiovascular changes in the mother, and blood flow to the breasts (and gastrointestinal tract and liver) is increased (Lawrence 1980). The discomfort that the mother experiences in the first 2–4 days after birth will depend on the extent of the increase. The early changes are not due to the breasts being overfull with milk (Ingelman-Sundberg 1953), and neither expression nor oxytocin administration is of value.

Milk engorgement

Since the initiation of the vascular changes in the breasts and the secretion of milk are both the result of the uninhibited action of prolactin, there is a degree of overlap between vascular engorgement and milk production. The milk, once secreted, is stored in the alveoli, which are surrounded by myoepithelial cells (see p. 23). When the baby is correctly attached to the breast, the oxytocin released by suckling causes these cells to contract and propel the milk forward into the lactiferous sinuses beneath the areola, where it can be removed by the baby. If the milk is not removed as it is formed – as regulated by the baby's need to go to the breast – either because the baby's access to the breast is restricted, or because of incorrect positioning once there, it is quite likely that as milk production rapidly increases the volume of milk in the breast will exceed the capacity of the alveoli to store it comfortably.

The longer the milk remains in the breast, the more the feedback inhibitor of lactation is able to build up and milk suppression will begin (see p. 27). The subsequent over-distension of the alveoli causes the milk-secreting cells to become flattened, drawn out and even to rupture (Dawson 1935), and further milk production begins to be suppressed. In some instances the pressure in the alveoli may be sufficiently high to force substances from the milk into the capillaries or connective tissues. This, in turn, will activate the mother's immune system – her pulse and temperature will rise, a red, painful area appears on the breast and the aching, flu-like feeling she experiences may be accompanied by rigors (Gunther 1973). These are the classical symptoms of non-infective mastitis which, if untreated, may progress to infective mastitis and even abscess formation (see below).

Prevention of engorgement

Milk engorgement is almost always iatrogenic: it rarely occurs when mothers are able to feed their babies 'on demand' day and night (Applebaum 1977, Fildes 1979, Thomsen et al 1984) (see pp. 65–66). It may be further prevented by ensuring that the baby is correctly attached on each occasion so that the milk is efficiently removed and the 'let-down' reflex effectively stimulated.

Treatment

If a breastfeeding woman develops milk engorgement, attention must first be paid to the possible cause. If the mother is attempting to regulate either the frequency or duration of the feeds she should be dissuaded from doing so. She may mistakenly believe that her baby must feed from both breasts at each feed (see p. 64). Her feeding technique should be observed and help given, if necessary, to ensure effective attachment

Sometimes the act of gentle hand expression to soften the breast by pushing away the oedema, prior to feeding, is all that is necessary. Some women find this easier to do in a warm shower or bath. In many instances this is sufficient, although sometimes gentle mechanical expression may also be helpful. Only if the engorgement has progressed to the point of inflammation may it be necessary to express milk gently after the feed (by hand or pump) until the engorgement has subsided (Thomsen et al 1984). Expressing in this context (i.e. to relieve engorgement) will not make the mother's breasts overproduce. The engorgement is the result of inefficent milk removal, not too much milk.

Cold compresses between feeds may also be comforting, although there is no evidence that this is generally effective.

Traditional home remedies include the application of raw cabbage leaves. The effectiveness of this treatment has been evaluated in one RCT (Nicodem et al 1994), which found no significant difference in the resolution of engorgement between the two groups. However, the study found that the use of cabbage leaves did no harm and might have a beneficial effect, even if it were psychological rather than purely physical.

Prevention and treatment of mastitis

The term 'mastitis' should not be regarded as synonymous with 'breast infection'. Although inflammation of the breast may be the result of an infective process, in over 50% of cases it is not

(Ingelman-Sundberg 1953, Lawrence 1980, Smith 1974). Thus automatic recourse to antibiotic therapy may be inappropriate.

Non-infective mastitis

If the milk is not removed from the breast at the rate at which it is produced, the pressure in the alveoli will start to rise. This rise may be generalised, as in the case of engorgement, or localised.

The commonest cause will be milk stasis secondary to poor attachment. It may also result from the baby suddenly having a much longer gap than usual between feeds. Rarely it may be the result of some specific internal or external obstruction (e.g. blocked duct, bruising from trauma or rough handling, compression from fingers holding the breast, or a tight brassiere). (Small 'lumps' in the breast are often referred to as blocked ducts, but they are usually due to localised inflammation rather than a physical obstruction.)

If the situation is not relieved, the pressure in the alveoli may become sufficiently high to cause milk substances to be forced out into the surrounding tissue (see p. 104).

Infective mastitis

Breast infections may occur in the outer skin of the breast, or within the glandular or connective tissue deeper in the breast. Unless this is treated quickly, abscess formation may take place.

Prevention of non-infective mastitis

This condition is often a consequence of engorgement, and should be prevented in the same way. Correct attachment is an essential part of the prevention of this condition.

Localised obstructions should be avoided by advising the woman not to wear clothing that puts pressure on her breasts, to handle her breasts gently to avoid bruising, not to grip her breast tightly when supporting it while feeding, and to treat any lumpiness in the breast promptly by encouraging drainage from that area, improving attachment and perhaps very gently stroking the affected area downward towards the nipple. Vigorous breast massage may make the situation worse if milk already under pressure in the alveoli is forced into the connective tissue.

Prevention of infective mastitis

The epithelium of the breast and nipple may be damaged by incorrect attachment of the baby at the breast, or occasionally by the use of creams, lotions or sprays to which the mother is sensitive and which subsequently damage the skin (Minchin 1998).

Bacterial infection requires that organisms breach the protective barrier of the skin and are able to multiply in spite of the body's defence system.

Unresolved non-infective mastitis may progress to infective mastitis (Thomsen et al 1984).

Treatment of mastitis

In the past any inflammation of the breast was likely to be treated with systemic antibiotics. This seems to be because it was not recognised that the inflammation was not necessarily caused by an infection (Inch & Fisher 1995, Marshall et al 1975, Neibyl et al 1978), and partly because then, as now, culturing milk samples took too long for the results to be used as the basis for starting treatment.

However, one study (Thomsen et al 1984) suggested that an effective differential diagnosis can be made on the basis of a leucocyte and bacterial count of samples of breast milk – a test that can be completed rapidly in a laboratory. The study found that women who were displaying the signs and symptoms of 'mastitis' but whose milk contained fewer than 10^6 leucocytes per mL and fewer than 10^3 bacteria per mL needed no treatment other than to continue breastfeeding. Those with fewer than 10^6 leucocytes but more than 10^3 bacteria per mL benefited from expressing milk after a feed as well as continuing to breastfeed. Only those with a leucocyte count in excess of 10^6 per mL and a bacterial count in excess of 10^3 per mL were deemed to be suffering from infective mastitis and required antibiotics in addition to breastfeeding and expressing after feeds.

Most antimicrobial drugs taken by the mother do not, in general, appear in her breast milk in amounts sufficient to affect her nursing infant (White & White 1984), although some adverse effects have been noted, principally rashes, diarrhoea and thrush (Brodie 1986). (These drugs may also produce similar side-effects in the mother.) Thus, it would be of benefit if, by employing some means of rapid differential diagnosis, such as a modification of that described above, the infant of a mother who developed breast inflammation was not, in consequence, automatically exposed to the possibility of such side-effects.

In the absence of this facility, provided it was possible to monitor the mother closely, it might be appropriate to delay antibiotic therapy for 12–24 h, whilst taking the corrective measures described above. If, however, there was no improvement during this time, a broad-spectrum antibiotic (such as cephalexin or flucloxacillin) would be necessary.

If it is not possible to provide close professional supervision and support for a mother with mastitis, prophylactic antibiotics will be needed from the outset. Finally, there is no justification for advising a lactating woman with mastitis to stop breastfeeding – indeed, abrupt weaning appears to increase the chances that the woman will develop a breast abscess (Marshall et al 1975) (see also p. 121).

The guidance below is abstracted from the World Health Organization (2000) publication 'Mastitis: causes and management' (see Further Reading). The main principles of treatment of mastitis are described below.

Supportive counselling

Mastitis is a painful and frustrating experience, and it makes many women feel very ill. In addition to effective treatment and control of pain, a woman needs emotional support. *She may have been given conflicting advice from health professionals, she may have been advised to stop breastfeeding, or she may have been given no guidance either way.* She may be confused and anxious, and unwilling to continue breastfeeding.

The woman needs reassurance about the value of breast-feeding: that it is safe to continue; that milk from the affected breast will not harm her infant; and that her breast will recover both its shape and function subsequently. She needs encouragement that it is worth the effort to overcome her current difficulties.

She needs clear guidance about all measures needed for treatment, and how to continue breastfeeding or expressing milk from the affected breast. She will need follow-up to give continuing support and guidance until she has recovered fully.

Effective milk removal
This is the most essential part of treatment. Antibiotics and symptomatic treatment may make a woman feel better temporarily, but unless milk removal is improved the condition may become worse or relapse despite the antibiotics.

- Help the mother to improve her infant's attachment at the breast.
- Encourage frequent breastfeeding, as often and as long as the infant is willing, without restrictions.
- If necessary, express breast milk by hand or with a pump, until breastfeeding can be resumed.

Antibiotic therapy
Antibiotic treatment is indicated if any of the following applies.

- symptoms do not improve after 12–24 h of improved milk removal
- cell and bacterial colony counts and culture are available and indicate infection
- symptoms have been present for a day or more and are increasing in severity.

An appropriate antibiotic must be used (Table 8.1). To be effective against *Staphylococcus aureus*, a β-lactamase-resistant antibiotic is needed. For Gram-negative organisms, cefalexin or amoxicillin may be the most appropriate. If possible, milk from the affected breast should be cultured and the antibiotic sensitivity of the bacteria determined.

Table 8.1 Antibiotics for the treatment of infective mastitis

Antibiotic	Dosage
Erythromycin	250–500 mg 6 hourly
Flucloxacillin	250 mg 6 hourly
Dicloxacillin	125–500 mg 6 hourly by mouth
Amoxicillin	250–500 mg every 8 h
Cefalexin	250–500 mg 6 hourly

The chosen antibiotic must be given for an adequate length of time: 10–14 days is now recommended by most authorities. Shorter courses are associated with a higher incidence of relapse.

Symptomatic treatment

Pain should be treated with an analgesic. Ibuprofen is considered the most effective, and it may help to reduce inflammation as well as pain. Paracetamol is an appropriate alternative.

Rest may be appropriate if the woman feels ill. As well as helping the woman herself, resting in bed with her infant is a useful way to increase the frequency of breastfeeds, and may thus improve milk removal.

Other measures that are recommended are the application of warm packs to the breast, which both relieves pain and helps the milk to flow, and ensuring that the woman drinks sufficient fluid.

References

Alexander J, Grant A, Campbell M. Randomised trial of breast shells and Hoffman's exercises for inverted and non-protractile nipples. BMJ 1992; 304:1030–1032.

Alper JC, Welch EA, Ginsberg M et al. Moist wound healing under a vapor permeable membrane. J Am Acad Dermatol 1983; 8(3):347–353.

Anonymous. Current concepts and approaches to wound healing. Crit Care Med 1988; 16(9).

Applebaum RM. The modern management of successful breastfeeding. Pediatr Clin North Am 1977; 241(1):37–47.

Beske EJ, Garvis MS. Important factors in breastfeeding success. Maternal and Child Nursing 1982; 7:174–179.

Brockway L. Hair colour and problems in breastfeeding. Midwives Chronicle and Nursing Notes 1986; March:66–67.

Brodie MJ. Drugs and breastfeeding. Practitioner 1986; 230: 483–485.

Brown MS, Hurlock JT. Preparation of the breast for breastfeeding. Nurs Res 1975; 24:448–451.

Carvalho M, Robertson S, Klaus M. Does the duration and frequency of early breastfeeding affect nipple pain? Birth 1984; 11(2):81–84.

Clark M. A study of 4 methods of nipple care offered to post partum mothers. N Z Nurs J 1985; 78:16–18.

Dawson EK. Edinb Med J 1935; 42:569.

Duffy EP, Percival P, Kershaw E. Positive effects of an antenatal group teaching session on postnatal nipple pain, nipple trauma and breastfeeding rates. Midwifery 1997; 13:189–196.

Fildes V. Putting mum in the picture. Nursing Mirror 1979; 149(3):22–24.

Freidman EA, Sachtleben MR. Oxytocin in lactation. Am J Obstet Gynecol 1961; 82:846–855.

Gans B. Breast and nipple pain in the early stages of lactation. BMJ 1958; 4 October:830–834.

Garcia J, Garforth S. A national study of policy and practice in midwifery. Oxford: National Perinatal Epidemiology Unit, Radcliffe Infirmary; 1985.

Goodine LA, Fried PA. Infant feeding practices: pre and post natal factors affecting choice of method and duration of breastfeeding. Can J Public Health 1984; 75:439–444.

Gueri M, Jutsum P, White A. Evaluation of a breastfeeding campaign in Trinidad. Bol Of Sanit Panam 1979; 86(3):189–195.

Gunther M. Sore nipples – cause and prevention. Lancet 1945; ii:590–593.

Gunther M. Infant feeding. Harmondsworth, UK: Penguin; 1973.

Herd B, Feeney JG. Two aerosol sprays in nipple trauma. Practitioner 1986; 230:31–38.

Hewat RJ, Ellis DJ. A comparison of the effectiveness of two methods of nipple care. Birth 1987; 41(1):41–45.

Hoddinott P, Pill R. Qualitative study of decisions about infant feeding among women in East End of London. BMJ 1999, 318(7175): 30–34.

Houston MJ. Learning to breastfeed (appendix). In: Minchin MK, ed. Breastfeeding matters. Australia: Allen & Unwin; 1985: 105–106.

Howie PW, McNeilly AS, McArdle T, Smart L, Houston MJ. The relationship between suckling induced prolactin response and lactogenesis. J Clin Endocrinol Metab 1980; 50:670–673.

Hytten FE. Clinical and chemical studies in lactation. IX. Breastfeeding in hospital. BMJ 1954; 18 December:1447–1452.

Inch S, Fisher C. Antiseptic sprays and nipple trauma. Practitioner 1987; 230:1037–1038.

Inch S, Fisher C. Mastitis in lactating women – infection or inflammation? Practitioner 1995; 239:472–476.

Ingelman-Sundberg A. Early puerperal engorgement. Acta Paediatr Scand 1953; 32:399–402.

Ingelman-Sundberg A. The value of antenatal massage of the nipples and expression of colostrum. Journal of Obstetrics and Gynaecology of the British Empire 1958; 65(3):448–449.

hnson CA, Garza C, Nichols B. A teaching intervention to improve breastfeeding success. J Nutr Educ 1984; 16:19–22.

Jones D. Breastfeeding problems. Nursing Times 1984; 80(33):53–54.

Kaplowitz DD. The effect of an education programme on the decision to breastfeed. J Nutr Educ 1983; 15:61–65.

Kirk TR. An evaluation of the impact of breastfeeding promotions in Edinburgh. Proc Nutr Soc 1979; 38:77A.

Ladas AK. The relationship of information and support to behavior, the La Leche League and breastfeeding. PhD dissertation, Columbia University, New York; 1970.

Lawrence R. Breastfeeding – a guide for the medical profession. St. Louis: CV Mosby; 1980.

L'Esperance CM. Pain or pleasure: the dilemma of early breastfeeding. Birth and the Family Journal 1980; 7(1):21–26.

Littman H, Medendorp SV, Goldfarb J. The decision to breastfeed: the importance of fathers' approval. Clin Pediatr 1994; 33(4): 214–219.

Mackey S, Fried PA. Infant breast and bottle-feeding practices: some related factors and attitudes. Can J Public Health 1981; 72:312–318.

MAIN Trial Collaborative Group. Preparing for breast feeding: treatment of inverted nipples and non-protractile nipples in pregnancy. Midwifery 1994; 10:200–214.

Marshall BR et al. Sporadic puerperal mastitis. JAMA 1975; 233(13):1377–1379.

Midwives Information and Resource Service/NHS Centre for Reviews and Dissemination. Feeding your baby: breast or bottle? Informed Choice leaflet no. 7. Bristol: MIDIRS and NHS Centre for Reviews and Dissemination 1999 (available from MIDIRS, 9 Elmdale Road, Bristol BS8 1SL, UK).

Minchin M. Breastfeeding matters. Australia: Allen & Unwin; 1998.

Neibyl JR et al. Sporadic (non epidemic) puerperal mastitis. J Reprod Med 1978; 20(2):97–100.

Newton N. Nipple pain and nipple damage. J Pediatr 1952; 41:411–423.

Nicholson W. Cracked nipples in breastfeeding mothers – a randomised trial of three methods of management. Newsletter of the Nursing Mothers of Australia 1985; 21(4):7–10.

Nicodem VC, Danziger D, Gebka N et al. Do cabbage leaves prevent engorgement? A RCT study. Birth 1994; 20:61–64.

Pugh LC, Buchko L, Bishop BA et al. A comparison of topical agents to relieve nipple pain and enhance breastfeeding. Birth 1996; 23(2):88–93.

Ruis H. Oxytocin enhances the onset of lactation amongst mothers delivering prematurely. BMJ 1981; 283:340–342.

Shurtz AR et al. Comparison of nipple care in the puerperium with powder and ointment. Gerburtshilfe Frauenheik 1978; 38:573–576.

Sjolin S, Hofvander Y, Hillervick C. A prospective study of individual courses of breastfeeding. Acta Paediatr Scand 1979; 68:521–529.

Slaven S, Harvey D. Unlimited sucking time improves breastfeeding. Lancet 1981; i:392–393.

Slaven S, Harvey D, Craft I. A double-blind controlled trial of chlorhexidine in aerosol spray for the prevention of sore nipples (unpublished results). Cited in: Inch S. Difficulties in breastfeeding – midwives in disarray? J R Soc Med 1987; 80:53–57.

Smith VR. The mammary gland – development and maintenance of lactation. Vol. 1. New York: Academic Press; 1974

Svejcar J. Methodological approaches to the promotion and maintenance of breastfeeding. Klin Pediatr 1977; 189:333–336.

Switzky LT, Vietze P, Switzky HN. Attitudinal and demographic predictors of breastfeeding and bottlefeeding behaviour by mothers of six week-old infants. Psychol Rep 1979; 45:3–14.

Thomsen AC et al. Course and treatment of milk stasis, non-infectious inflammation of the breast and infectious mastitis in nursing women. Am J Obstet Gynecol 1984; 149(5):492–495.

Waller H, Aschaffenburg R, Grant MW. Biochem J 1941; 35:272.

White A, Freeth S, O'Brien M. Infant feeding 1990. London: HMSO; 1992.

White GJ, White M. Breastfeeding and drugs in human milk. Vet Hum Toxicol 1984; 26(Suppl 1):3.

Whitley N. Preparation of the breasts for breastfeeding. A one year follow-up of 34 mothers. J Obstet Gynecol Neonatal Nurs 1978; 7(3):44–48.

Wiles LS. The effect of prenatal breastfeeding education on breastfeeding success and maternal perception of the infant. J Obstet Gynaecol Neonatal Nurs 1984; 13:253–257.

Winter GD, Scales JT. The effect of air drying and dressings on the surface of a wound. Nature 1963; 5 January:91–92.

Woolridge MW, Baum D, Drewett RF. Effect of a traditional and of a new nipple shield on sucking patterns and milk flow. Early Hum Dev 1980; 4(4):357–364.

Zinaman MJ et al. Acute prolactin and oxytocin responses and milk yield to infant suckling and artifical methods of expression in lactating women. Pediatrics 1992; 89(3):437–440.

ʲurther Reading

World Health Organization. Mastitis: causes and management. WHO/FCH/CAH/00.13. Geneva: WHO, Department of Child and Adolescent Health and Development; 2000.

Notes on less common problems

Baby vomiting blood or digested blood in stools   115
Blood in milk or colostrum   115
Blanching of the nipple (white nipple)   116
Thrush infection   116
Contact dermatitis   117
Diabetes   117
Epilepsy   117
Anticoagulant therapy   117
Other drugs and breastfeeding   117
Mammary surgery   118
Cleft lip   118
Cleft palate   118
Down syndrome   119
Tandem feeding   119
Breast abscess   119
Inverted nipples   119
HIV and breastfeeding   120
Hepatitis B   121
Hepatitis C   121
Herpes simplex infection   121

Baby vomiting blood or digested blood in stools

Blood in vomited breast milk or in stools (*melaena spuria*) often originates from a damaged nipple. Breastfeeding should continue and the cause of the damage should be corrected (see pp. 101–104). If the diagnosis is uncertain, blood can be tested for adult or fetal haemoglobin. The stool can be tested for blood to distinguish digested blood from meconium.

Blood in milk or colostrum

This condition occurs infrequently and appears to be harmless. The cause is unclear, but it may be due to leakage of blood through the tight junctions of the cells lining the alveoli. It usually resolves spontaneously as the milk 'comes in' and breast-feeding should not be interrupted. However, if the condition persists or the mother is anxious, it would seem prudent to seek informed medical opinion.

Blanching of the nipple (white nipple)

This painful condition may be associated with circulatory problems, such as Raynaud phenomenon (intermittent ischaemia secondary to vasospasm). Attachment of the baby should be checked as trauma or mechanical compression seems to trigger this response. Helpful reported remedies include keeping the breasts warm, feeding in a warmer room and drinking tea (which contains the vasodilator theophylline) before the feed.

Severe cases may respond favourably to nifedipine, but treatment may take several weeks to be effective (Lawlor-Smith & Lawlor-Smith 1996, 1997).

Thrush infection

This is an occasional cause of sore nipples, although the incidence seems to be increasing, as it is more common in women who have been treated with antibiotics (Amir 1991). Thrush infection can be distinguished from the soreness caused by poor attachment by observation of feeding technique; also, it often occurs after a period of trouble-free feeding. It commonly occurs bilaterally and may appear evenly distributed around the base of the nipple and possibly the part of the areola most in contact with the baby's mouth while feeding. The nipple pain intensifies during the feed and continues for some time between feeds. The nipple and areola are often pink and shiny, and may be moist. In some cases the baby may also have clinically obvious oral or perianal thrush.

If thrush is suspected, both the mother and her baby should be treated simultaneously with topical preparations (e.g. creams, oral gels and suspensions) to prevent reinfection. (Clotrimazole (Canésten) should be avoided as it may cause skin irritation on the breast and nipple.) The mother is more likely to tolerate the discomfort when she knows there is a cure.

Very rarely the lactiferous ducts may also become infected, giving rise to deep breast pain. In such cases systemic treatment will be needed (Lawrence 1994). Poor technique and nipple thrush may coexist.

Contact dermatitis

Women may develop dermatitis of the nipple and breast from unpurified lanolin or other ointments, from chlorhexidine spray or from detergents in brassieres. All local applications should be stopped. If it is likely that the dermatitis is caused by the woman's bra, she should use breast pads that are not plastic backed and wash her clothing in soap. Treatment with hydrocortisone 0.5%, under medical direction, may be indicated (Gunther 1973).

Diabetes

This is not a contraindication to breastfeeding. If the mother is insulin dependent her regimen will be adjusted as part of her routine treatment. Her intention to breastfeed must be conveyed to her physician as she may require less insulin (Miller 1977, Whichelow & Doddridge 1983).

Epilepsy

Drugs that are considered safe for pregnancy will be safe for breastfeeding, as they are more likely to pass the placental barrier than to be excreted in milk. If the mother is prone to seizures she should feed where the baby will come to no harm. (The breastfed baby is certainly at no greater risk than the bottle-fed one in such situations and, as a breastfeeding mother can lie down to feed, her baby may be at less risk.)

Anticoagulant therapy

Heparin and warfarin may safely be given while breastfeeding (L'E Orme et al 1977). Expert advice should be sought for other drugs.

Other drugs and breastfeeding

Most health authorities and health boards have a drug information centre that will help with any enquiries about maternal medication during lactation. Otherwise, hospital pharmacies should be able to obtain the necessary information. In the case of commonly used drugs it is unlikely that the risks to the baby outweigh the benefits of breastfeeding. In almost all cases, a safer alternative drug can be found, or at worst breastfeeding need be interrupted only briefly (Wilson 1981). (See also Further reading, p. 123.)

Mammary surgery

Women can breastfeed successfully following unilateral mastectomy, provided the other breast is functionally normal. Women who have had silicone implants or reduction mammoplasty may be able to breastfeed successfully as it is probable that both the nerve supply to the nipple and the ductal system necessary for sustained lactation will have been left intact in these cases. If the nipple has been resited, it is most unlikely that breastfeeding will be possible.

Cleft lip

Cleft lip should not cause any breastfeeding problems. Some surgeons encourage breastfeeding soon after plastic surgery; others advise an initial period of spoon-feeding.

Cleft palate

This defect causes major problems. The baby cannot create a seal between his mouth and the breast and cannot therefore make a teat out of the breast and nipple, which is the prerequisite of efficient milk removal. The defect can be 'closed' with a feeding plate or palate seal, but even with this most babies still have great difficulty breastfeeding. It appears that the sucking reflex is most effectively stimulated by the sensation of the nipple against the baby's palate (Gunther 1955, Peiper 1963) and the stimulus is thus greatly reduced with this condition. Mothers who want to feed their babies with their own milk can do so by expressing their breast milk and feeding it to the baby with a special bottle, teat or spoon. Breastfeeding can be attempted, and may even be successful if the mother has large, elastic breasts and a ready milk ejection reflex, but it is usually necessary to supplement while breastfeeding with a nursing supplementer (Danner 1986).

Down syndrome

These babies need extra help during the initiation period, and much time and patience is required to ensure that they are properly attached to the breast at each feed. The mother may need to express her milk while this learning process is proceeding. The benefits of breastfeeding assume particular importance for these babies.

Tandem feeding

Midwives may occasionally encounter a mother who continues to breastfeed throughout her subsequent pregnancy, and breastfeeds both the newborn baby and his sibling afterwards. There is no evidence to suggest that this is harmful for the mother or her children. It is important, however, that the newborn baby's needs are met first. (In practice many young children cease feeding during the mother's pregnancy. It is suggested that the volume reduces and the taste changes.) Nipple tenderness is commonly reported by mothers who breastfeed during pregnancy.

Breast abscess

Abscess formation requires that pathogens breach the protective barrier of the skin and multiply in spite of the body's defence system. Abscesses may form superficially, often near the areola, or deep within the substance of the breast. These deeper abscesses are often the result of unresolved non-infective mastitis which has damaged the tissues and made them vulnerable to infection. Once an abscess has formed, it may be necessary to incise the breast in order to drain it. Unless the position of the incision makes it impossible, breastfeeding should continue as this is likely to speed healing (Benson & Goodman 1970). Alternatively, the abscess may be aspirated, which avoids the necessity for hospital admission (Dixon 1988). Feeding should continue uninterrupted on the unaffected side and the baby returned to the affected side as quickly as possible.

Inverted nipples

Although uncommon, inverted nipples present a real challenge to midwives. There is now evidence that neither Woolwich shells nor the use of the Hoffman technique is beneficial (MAIN Trial Collaborative Group 1994). Nipple shape (or lack of nipple) is less important than the protractility of the surrounding tissue, as it is this that determines the baby's ability to make an effective 'teat' from the breast (Gunther 1955).

No prediction of the ultimate success of breastfeeding should be made on the basis of antenatal inspection of a woman's nipples, as dramatic changes in shape often take place around parturition (see p. 33). If the midwife is initially unable to attach the baby to the breast effectively, lactation can be initiated and sustained with a breast pump, and further attempts made when the milk is 'in' and the breasts have softened.

Skilled help with attaching the baby in the first few days is particularly helpful in these cases. (See also p. 51.)

In 1994 a thimble-shaped device that was introduced to provide a non-surgical method of correcting inverted nipples in non-pregnant women began to be offered for sale commercially and was aimed at pregnant as well as non-pregnant women. Before being marketed, 19 (self-selected) women were 'treated' with the device, only three of whom were pregnant. Treatment consisted of giving the women the device and showing them how to use it (the device is placed over the nipple and the air withdrawn by means of a syringe). The length of time for which they wore it varied; no accurate records were kept. There was no control group. There was some evidence, even from this very small number, that the device could cause nipple damage, as two of the women, at least one of whom was pregnant, bled from their nipples as a result of the treatment (Inch & Fisher 1994). There is currently no basis on which this device can be recommended to pregnant women.

HIV and breastfeeding

Guidance concerning breastfeeding by women at risk of infection with human immunodeficiency virus (HIV) and amplification of the guidance on human milk banking is contained in a Department of Health letter 'HIV infection, breastfeeding and human milk banking in the United Kingdom' (PL/CMO(89)4; PL/CNO(89)3) and in the national milk banking guidelines (Royal College of Paediatrics and Child Health & UK Association for Milk Banking 1999). Women who are HIV antibody positive should be advised that it is prudent to avoid breastfeeding (RCM 1998). Women who are at risk of HIV infection and are HIV negative or decline serotesting should receive counselling. Some may need to be advised about the risks of transmission as if they were HIV positive. Serotesting should be made available.

Hepatitis B

All babies born to mothers who are known to be hepatitis B positive should be vaccinated at birth. If the mother is E antigen positive she is highly infectious; her baby should receive immunoglobulin and she should be advised not to breastfeed (Royal College of Paediatrics and Child Health & UK Association for Milk Banking 1999).

If the mother is E antibody positive (in common with 80% of the population), she is not infectious and can breastfeed safely. If she is negative to both E antigen and E antibodies, she and her baby should be treated as if infectious.

Hepatitis C

Much less is currently known about the risks associated with breast-feeding if the mother is hepatitis C positive. It is at present unclear whether hepatitis C can be transmitted in breast milk (Koff 1992).

Herpes simplex infection

If a mother has a lesion on her breast, it should be regarded as infectious for the first 5 days (Spruance et al 1977). During this time the baby may be at risk of infection if fed directly from the breast. If this is thought to be the case, milk should be expressed (to maintain lactation) and the expressed milk fed to the baby after a few hours have elapsed, using a spoon or bottle. (Since the mother will have been infectious before the lesion developed, her milk will contain antibodies to the virus. These will remain in the milk after expression and afford some measure of protection for the baby. Allowing a few hours to elapse between expressing the milk and giving it to the baby may mean a lowered level of the virus in the milk as a result of its antiviral properties (Cerutti & White 1981).)

If the lesion is not on the breast, and the baby is not likely to come into direct contact with it, breastfeeding may continue, but the mother should be advised to pay particular attention to washing her hands before feeding her baby (Yeager et al 1983).

References

Amir L. Candida and the lactating breast:predisposing factors. J Hum Lactation 1991; 7(4):177–181.

Benson EA, Goodman MA. An evaluation of the use of stilboestrol and antibiotics in the early management of acute puerperal breast abscess. Br J Surg 1970; 57:258.

Cerutti E, White G. Management of mother infant problems during lactation. Taped at the LLL physicians' seminar 1981 (available from La Leche League; for address see Appendix 1).

Danner SC. Breastfeeding your cleft lip/palate baby. Lactation Consultant Series. New Jersey: Avery Press; 1986 (or pamphlet available from Birth and Life Bookstore, PO Box 70625, Seattle, WA 98107, USA).

Department of Health. HIV infection, breastfeeding and human milk banking in the United Kingdom. PL/CMO(89)4; PL/CNO(89)3). London: HMSO; 1989. (Available from Health Publications Unit, No. 2 Site, Heywood, Lancashire OL10 2PZ, UK.)

Dixon JM. Repeated aspiration of breast abscess in lactating women. BMJ 1988; 10 December:1517–1518.

Gunther M. Instinct and the nursing couple. Lancet 1955; i:575–578.

Gunther M. Infant feeding. London: Penguin; 1973.

Inch S, Fisher C. The Avent Niplette – is it of value? AIMS Journal 1994; 5(4):13–14.

Koff RS. The low efficiency of maternal-neonatal transmission of hepatitis C virus: how certain are we? Ann Intern Med 1992; 117:967–969.

Lawlor-Smith L, Lawlor-Smith C. Nipple vasospasm in the breastfeeding woman. Breastfeeding Review 1996; 4(1):37–38.

Lawlor-Smith L, Lawlor-Smith C. Vasospasm of the nipple – a manifestation of Raynaud's phenomenon: case reports. BMJ 1997; 314:644–645.

Lawrence R. Breastfeeding – a guide for the medical profession. St Louis: Mosby; 1994.

L'E Orme M, Lewis PJ, de Swiet M et al. May mothers given warfarin breastfeed their infants? BMJ 1977; 18 June:1564–1565.

MAIN Trial Collaborative Group. Preparing for breast feeding: treatment of inverted nipples and non-protractile nipples in pregnancy. Midwifery 1994; 10:200–214.

Miller DL. Birth and long term unsupplemented breastfeeding in 17 insulin dependent mothers. Birth and the Family Journal 1977; 4:65–70.

Peiper A. Cerebral function in infancy and childhood. 3rd edn. New York: Consultants Bureau; 1963:418–420.

Royal College of Midwives. HIV and AIDS. RCM position paper number 16a. London: Royal College of Midwives; 1998.

Royal College of Paediatrics and Child Health & UK Association for Milk Banking. Guidelines for the establishment and operation of human milk banks in the UK. 2nd edn. London: Royal College of Paediatrics and Child Health & UK Association for Milk Banking; 1999.

Spruance SL, Overall JC, Kern ER et al. The natural history of recurrent herpes simplex labialis. N Engl J Med 1977; 297(2):57–70.

Whichelow MJ, Doddridge MC. Lactation in diabetic women. BMJ 1983; 287:649.

Wilson JT. Drugs in breastmilk. Lancaster: MTP; 1981.

Yeager AS, Ashley RL, Corey L. Transmission of herpes simplex virus from father to neonate. J Pediatr 1983; 103(6):905–907.

Further reading

Hale T. Medications and mothers' milk. Amarillo, TX: Pharmasoft Medical Publishing; 1998.

Lee A, Inch S, Finnagan D (eds). Therapeutics in pregnancy and lactation. Oxford: Radcliffe Medical Press, 2000.

Breastfeeding under special circumstances

Preterm infants	124
HIV and milk banking	125
Caesarean section	126
Twins	126
Triplets	127
Establishing lactation with an electric pump	127
Alternatives to bottle-feeding	130
Babies being cared for in units other than maternity units	131

One of the midwife's main roles is to ensure that women who wish to lactate and breastfeed do so successfully. In circumstances where the mother is under additional pressure or the normal mechanisms for ensuring successful lactation are interrupted, the mother will need particular help. In neonatal intensive and special care units, for example, the nursing priority may be to ensure that the baby makes rapid progress and is speedily discharged.

Sometimes, these objectives, with their emphasis on tube feeding and/or preterm formula, may be at odds with establishment of the mother's lactation. Once the child is returned to his mother's care, it is she who will be solely responsible for his nutrition, and it would be regrettable if the opportunity for long-term breastfeeding was sacrificed at an early stage in favour of short-term gains. Midwives should do all they can to protect the mother's lactation in these circumstances.

Preterm infants

For mothers who have successfully initiated lactation with an electric pump, the transition from tube feeds to breastfeeding can be very difficult. The preterm tube-fed baby is deprived of the sucking and swallowing experiences he has had in utero, and so may be artificially delayed in his competence at feeding. If he has received his mother's milk by bottle, he may need help adapting his feeding technique, and his mother will need particularly caring support at this time.

Babies are naturally equipped for feeding at the breast, so once they are developmentally competent they should not be denied the opportunity to feed on the grounds that it would be 'too tiring'. It has been demonstrated (Berbaum et al 1982) that preterm infants who are able to suck find breastfeeding less stressful than bottle-feeding.

Two studies have also shown that preterm infants allowed intermittent sucking on a 'blind teat' gained weight more rapidly than those who were not. It is possible that sucking facilitates the utilisation of tube-fed milk (Field et al 1982, Meier & Cranston-Anderson 1987). (This may be due to release of lingual lipase during sucking.) Allowing preterm infants to suckle at their mother's breast as soon as they are able would therefore be of benefit to both the baby and the mother.

Babies are neurologically and developmentally competent to suck and swallow at 32 weeks' gestation, and experience at breastfeeding may aid maturation of the process. However, attempting to provide sucking experience with either a bottle teat or a dummy may be detrimental to some in the long term, as the techniques required for feeding from a breast and a bottle are different from each other (see p. 42).

Babies as small as 1300–1400 g can breastfeed successfully (Meier & Cranston-Anderson 1987) if hospital staff are well informed and hospital structures supportive. Excellent reviews of the problems of feeding low-birthweight babies are available free of charge from the World Health Organization (Distribution and Sales Service, 1211 Geneva 27, Switzerland, or by mail order from HMSO Publications Centre, 51 Nine Elms Lane, London SW8 5DR, UK).

HIV and milk banking

Donor breast milk has a variety of important uses, ranging from the early feeds of the very small preterm (24–28 weeks) who seem to tolerate breast milk better than any other milk (Lucas 1987), to avoiding the use of cow's milk on the rare occasions when a breastfed baby is temporarily unable to take the breast.

Although concern about the possibility of the spread of HIV through the use of donor milk resulted in the closure of many milk banks, research strongly suggests that pasteurisation eliminates any risk of the transmission of HIV (Eglin & Wilkinson 1987).

Guidance issued by the Chief Medical Officer and endorsed by the Department of Health's Expert Advisory Group on AIDS recommends that women at risk of HIV infection should not donate milk intended for other women's babies.

Women willing to donate should be given an explanatory leaflet about the reasons for self-exclusion by women at risk and the significance of the HIV test. An HIV antibody test must be performed and a negative result received before the donor's milk can be accepted (Department of Health 1989, Royal College of Paediatrics and Child Health & UK Association for Milk Banking 1999). Potential donors should be reassured that the Association of British Insurers has stated that milk donors will not be affected in their application for life insurance or mortgages if they have been tested for HIV as a result of a milk bank screening procedure (Royal College of Paediatrics and Child Health & UK Association for Milk Banking 1999).

There are currently (in 2001) 14 human milk banks in the UK. In 1997 the UK Association of Milk Banks (Queen Charlotte's and Chelsea Hospital, London; tel: 020 8383 3559) was set up to support existing milk banks and to encourage the setting up of new ones.

Caesarean section

There is no evidence to support the long-established belief that caesarean section itself has any deleterious effect on the establishment of lactation. The mother will probably require more help to find a comfortable feeding position and attaching the baby to the breast in the first few days than she would if she had been vaginally delivered (Lewis et al 1980).

Twins

Nature is generous, and initially most women have a milk supply that is sufficient to feed two babies. Provided that both babies feed well, there will continue to be enough for both. The mother should be encouraged to feed each baby individually

during the early days so that the common early problem
resolved efficiently. Each baby may have its own breast,
may be switched at each feed. Some mothers will prefer to
tinue feeding the babies separately, some prefer to feed t
simultaneously, and some will adapt according to the babies'
natural feeding pattern (Saint et al 1986) (see also Appendix 2).

Triplets

There are many recorded cases of triplets being successfully
breastfed, but it requires a very committed mother and a lot of
extra help and support (MacDonald 1982).

Establishing lactation with an electric pump

There is little similarity between the action of a breast pump and
the action of a baby feeding at the breast. It is also known that
less prolactin is released when a breast pump is used than when
the baby feeds directly (Howie 1985).

In spite of this, many women succeed in initiating lactation
with a breast pump. However, unless the baby is able to start
feeding directly during the second or third week of life, the supply may begin to diminish, possibly as a result of falling prolactin
levels (Howie 1985). It is therefore of particular importance
that further suppression does not occur as a result of engorgement, and that the mother be encouraged to express milk as frequently (and as efficiently) as possible (Howie et al 1980).

As with breastfeeding, no specific timing restrictions should
be imposed on the length of each session, and the mother
should be encouraged to continue as long as a reasonable volume can be obtained; she should avoid pressing the funnel too
hard against the breast. It may also be helpful to support the
breast from beneath. However, unlike breastfeeding, it may be
beneficial to switch from side to side during the session.

Recent research conducted at North Staffordshire Hospital
suggests that gentle breast massage followed by double pumping (i.e. pumping both breasts at the same time) is the most
effective way of initiating and maintaining lactation (E. Jones,
personal communication).

Occasional breastfeeds should also be encouraged, if possible,
as these will help to maintain the supply.

The mother should be reassured that the pump is less efficient than a baby at milking the breast, and that she may well be capable of producing more milk than she can obtain by pumping.

In some circumstances, hand expression may be more appropriate or acceptable, and there is evidence to suggest that this technique results in higher prolactin levels (Howie 1985).

There are also several designs of hand pump available which are quite adequate once lactation is established but, as they are more tiring to use and less efficient than expression by hand or by electric pump expression, initiating lactation with a hand pump may be more difficult than with the other two methods.

Midwives should be aware that breast pumps are a potential source of infection (Moloney et al 1987). Mothers should be given sterile tubing (and if appropriate, 'safety' bottles) on each occasion that they use the pump and should be carefully instructed in its use. (On some older models it is necessary to take particular care to prevent milk entering the interior of the pump, and the collecting bottle in use with the model must be clearly marked to indicate the maximum permissible volume.) A record should be kept of all pump users and the pumps should be examined bacteriologically at regular intervals.

How to help a mother to express using an electric pump

Suggest that she:

1. Sits comfortably, with her back straight.
2. Supports her breast from underneath, with her fingers flat on her ribs and her index finger at the junction of her breast and ribs. This raises her breast tissue and allows it to be drawn easily into the funnel.
3. Ensures that her nipple is central in the funnel.
4. Keeps the funnel close enough to her breast to maintain the vacuum, but does not press it too firmly on to the breast or the breast tissue will be squashed.
5. Is patient – it often takes a minute or two for the milk to flow well.
6. Is guided by the milk flow, not the clock. Advise her to pump until the milk flow slows, and then switch to the second breast. When the flow slows on the second breast she can go

back to the first, and finally finish off on the second breast when the flow slows for the second time.

7. Pumps both breasts at the same time (double pumping) once she has got used to using the pump. If she is doing so, suggest that she turn the pump off for 30 seconds or so when the flow slows, and then turn it back on and continue until it slows down again. This seems to be more effective than pumping continuously.

Silicone inserts for pump collection kits

Some pump manufacturers supply a flexible insert or shield with the collecting kit. This will have the effect of reducing the internal diameter of the funnel. The mother should be advised to try the pump with and without the insert to discover which works better for her.

If the mother has a very broad nipple, the standard funnel will rub it and cause pain and damage. Larger funnels are available from some pump manufacturers. If larger funnels are not available, the mother will find hand expression less traumatic.

Storage of breast milk or colostrum

Provided it has been collected in a sterile container, breast milk is safe:

- at room temperature for up to 6 h (Ajusi et al 1989, Barger & Bull 1987, Larson et al 1984, Nwankwo et al 1988, Pittard et al 1985)
- in the fridge for up to 48 h, after which it can be frozen (Berkow et al 1984, Jensen & Jensen 1992).

It can remain frozen:

- in the ice box of a fridge for 1 week
- in a three-star freezer for up to 3 months.

Breast milk can be thawed overnight in the fridge or more quickly in a jug of warm water. The milk should not be given cold, but need not be warmer than room temperature before it is given to the baby. A microwave should not be used to thaw or heat milk (Nemethy & Clore 1990, Quan et al 1992).

whether fresh or thawed, that has been in contact
..the infant's saliva must be discarded if unused during a
...ding.

Alternatives to bottle-feeding

If it is necessary to give a breastfed baby his mother's milk
by some means other than directly from the breast, this can
be accomplished by a variety of methods: syringe, dropper,
spoon, cup, bottle or soft-spouted beaker, depending on the
age of the baby and the reason for not breastfeeding.

Baby-Friendly Hospitals should encourage the use of cups,
and this would seem appropriate for one or two feeds if given
to very young babies who only need small amounts, as it allows the
baby to remain more in control of his intake and thus consume
only what he needs. There is evidence that preterm babies can
cupfeed before they are able to suck, and thus cup-feeding can be
used as alternative to tube-feeding (Lang et al 1994).

Cup-feeding has now been extended as an alternative to
bottle-feeding breast milk to preterm infants in some neonatal
units. However, for longer-term use (particularly if the mother is expressing milk for her term baby to maintain her milk
supply and ensure adequate nutrition for the baby while she
deals with the problem of poor or difficult attachment), a
feeding bottle may be more satisfactory. It is quicker and less
wasteful than cup-feeding and, in most cases, more acceptable
to the mother.

There is currently concern that if a baby feeds from a bottle
he will somehow not be able to feed from a breast. This is often
referred to as 'nipple confusion'. There is no evidence to support this concern (Neifert et al 1995, Fisher & Inch 1996).
Several studies have now demonstrated that, if extra fluids are
given to breastfed babies, it makes no difference to the duration
of breastfeeding whether these are given by cup, cup and spoon,
or bottle and teat (Brown et al 1999, Cronenwett et al 1992,
Schubiger et al 1997).

There are undoubtedly conditions that may make it difficult
for the baby to make an effective teat from the breast; but these
difficulties are likely to be evident whether or not the baby is
given a bottle-feed.

Babies being cared for in units other than maternity units

There may be special circumstances in which babies are cared for in units without midwives being present (e.g. neonatal surgical unit, paediatric ward). Midwives should consider how best to give support to those mothers who wish to breastfeed.

References

Ajusi JD, Onyango FE, Mutanda LN et al. Bacteriology of unheated expressed milk stored at room temperature. East Afr Med J 1989; 66:381–387.

Barger J, Bull P. A comparison of the bacterial composition of breast-milk stored at room temperature and stored in the refrigerator. Int J Childbirth Educ 1987; August:29 30.

Berbaum J, Periera G, Peckham G. Increased oxygenation with non-nutritive sucking during gavage feeding in premature infants. Pediatr Res 1982; 16:278A.

Berkow S, Freed L, Hamosh M et al. Lipases and lipids in human milk: effect of freeze–thawing and storage. Pediatr Res 1984; 18:1257–1262.

Brown S, Alexander J, Thomas P. Feeding outcome in breastfed term babies supplemented by cup or bottle. Midwifery 1999; 15:92–96.

Cronenwett L, Stukel T, Kearney M et al. Single daily bottle use in the early weeks postpartum and breastfeeding outcomes. Pediatrics 1992; 90(5):760–766.

Davies M, Denton J. Feeding twins, triplets and more. London: Multiple Births Foundation, Queen Charlotte's and Chelsea Hospital; 1998.

Department of Health. HIV infection, breastfeeding and human milk banking in the UK. (PL/CMO(89)4; PL/CNO(89)3). London: HMSO; 1989 (available from: Health Publications Unit, No. 2 Site, Heywood OL10 2PZ, UK).

Eglin RP, Wilkinson AR. HIV infection and pasteurisation of breast-milk. Lancet 1987; i:1093.

Field T, Ignatoff E, Tringer S et al. Non-nutritive sucking during tube feedings: effects on preterm neonates in an intensive care unit. Pediatrics 1982; 70:381–384.

Fisher C, Inch S. Nipple confusion – who is confused? J Pediatr 1996;127:174.

Howie PJ. Breastfeeding – a new understanding. Midwives Chronicle and Nursing Notes 1985; July:184–192.

Howie PJ, McNeilly AS, McArdle T, Smart L, Houston MJ. The relationship between suckling-induced prolactin response and lactogenesis. J Clin Endocrinol Metab 1980; 50:670–673.

Jensen R, Jensen G. Specialty lipids for infant nutrition. 1. Milks and formulas. J Pediatr Gastroenterol Nutr 1992; 15:232–245.

Lang S, Lawrence CJ, Orme R. Cup feeding: an alternative method of infant feeding. Arch Dis Child 1994; 71:365–369.

Larson E, Zuill R, Zier V et al. Storage of human breast milk. Infect Control 1984; 5:127–130.

Lewis PJ, Devenish C, Kahn C. Controlled trial of metoclopramide in the initiation of breastfeeding. Br J Clin Pharmacol 1980; 9:217–219.

Lucas A. AIDS and human milk bank closures. Lancet 1987; i:1092–1093.

MacDonald D. More than one. Hornchurch, UK: Ian Henry Publications; 1982.

Meier P, Cranston-Anderson J. Responses of small preterm infants to bottle and breast-feeding. Maternal and Child Nursing 1987; 12:97–105.

Moloney AC, Quoraishi AH, Parry P, Hall V. A bacteriological examination of breast pumps. J Hosp Infect 1987; 9:169–174.

Neifert M, Lawrence R, Seacat J. Nipple confusion: towards a formal definition. J Pediatr 1995; 126:125–129.

Nemethy M, Clore ER. Microwave heating of infant formula and breastmilk. J Pediatr Health Care 1990; 4:131–135.

Nwankwo MU, Offor E, Okolo AA et al. Bacterial growth in expressed breastmilk. Ann Trop Paediatr 1988; 8:92–95.

Pittard WB, Anderson DM, Cerutti ER et al. Bacteriostatic qualities of human milk. J Pediatr 1985; 107:240–243.

Quan R, Yang C, Rubinstein S et al. Effects of microwave radiation on anti-infective factors in human milk. Pediatrics 1992; 89:667–669.

Royal College of Paediatrics and Child Health & UK Association for Milk Banking. Guidelines for the establishment and operation of human milk banks in the UK. 2nd edn. London: Royal College of Paediatrics and Child Health & UK Association for Milk Banking; 1999.

Saint L, Maggiore P, Hartmann PE. Yield and nutrient content of milk in 8 women breastfeeding twins and 1 woman breastfeeding triplets. Br J Nutr 1986; 56:49–58.

Schubiger G, Schwartz U, Tonz O. UNICEF/WHO Baby Friendly Initiative: does the use of bottles and pacifiers in the neonatal nursery prevent successful breastfeeding? Eur J Pediatr 1997; 156:874–877.

Further reading

United Kingdom Association for Milk Banking (UKAMB). Guidelines for the collection, storage and handling of breast milk for a mother's own baby on a neonatal unit. 2nd edn. London, UKAMB; 2001 (available from UKAMB, Queen Charlotte's and Chelsea Hospital, Du Cane Road, London W12 0HS).

Appendix I: The Ten Steps to Successful Breastfeeding

Every facility providing maternity services and care for newborn infants should:

1. Have a written breastfeeding policy that is routinely communicated to all healthcare staff.
2. Train all healthcare staff in the skills necessary to implement the breastfeeding policy.
3. Inform all pregnant women about the benefits and management of breastfeeding.
4. Help mothers to initiate breastfeeding within half an hour of giving birth.
5. Show mothers how to breastfeed and how to maintain lactation even if they are separated from their infants.
6. Give newborn infants no food or drink other than breast milk, unless medically indicated.
7. Practise rooming-in, allowing mothers and infants to remain together for 24 h a day.
8. Encourage breastfeeding on demand.
9. Give no artificial teats or pacifiers (also called dummies or soothers) to breastfeeding infants.
10. Foster the establishment of breastfeeding support groups and refer mothers to them on discharge from hospital or clinic.

Appendix 2: National and international voluntary organisations

National voluntary organisations

In many areas, traditional family support systems no longer exist, so that mothers are isolated. Where extended families still exist, support may come at the price of inaccurate information about breastfeeding. Midwives can help mothers to find a network of friends by giving them the addresses of the following organisations.

National Childbirth Trust
Breastfeeding Promotion Group
Alexandra House, Oldham Terrace
Acton
London W3 6NH
UK
Tel: 020 8992 8637

Breastfeeding Network
PO Box 11126
Paisley PA2 8YB
UK
Tel: 0870 900 8787
(this number will put the caller straight through to the nearest Network Supporter)

Twins and Multiple Births Association
41 Fortuna Way
Grimsby
South Humberside DN37 9SJ
UK

La Leche League (Great Britain)
Breastfeeding Help and Information
BM 3424
London WC1V 6XX
UK
Tel: 0207 242 1278

Baby Milk Action
6 Regent Terrace
Cambridge CB2 1AA
UK
Tel: 01223 464420

Association of Breastfeeding Mothers
7 Maybourne Close
Springfield Road
London SE26 6HQ
UK
Tel: 020 8676 0965

These organisations also supply information in accordance with these guidelines, by phone (24 hours a day, 7 days a week) and in leaflets and books. Their free leaflets contain useful information, and also include local and national contact addresses.

Midwives can assist by handing these leaflets to women antenatally, who can then make friends among the community of local mothers, and inform themselves about common breastfeeding problems and how to overcome them.

Before they leave the ward, mothers may appreciate receiving leaflets or cards giving details about the support organisations.

International voluntary organisations

Internationally, breastfeeding support and action organisations can be located by writing to:

GIFA (Geneva Infant Feeding Association)/IBFAN Europe
PO Box 157
1211 Geneva 19
Switzerland
(publishes breastfeeding briefs; useful update service)

IBFAN (International Baby Food Action Network) Africa
PO Box 34308
Nairobi
Kenya

Action for Corporate Accountability
910 17th Street

NW Suite 413
Washington, DC 20006
USA
Tel: 001 202 776 0595
(publishes IBFAN News)

LLLI (La Leche League International)
1400 North Meachan Road
Schaumburg
IL 60168
USA
Tel: 001 847 519 7730
(free catalogue; publishes breastfeeding abstracts)

IOCU (International Organisation of Consumer Unions)
PO Box 1045
Penang
Malaysia

NMAA (Nursing Mothers' Association of Australia)
PO Box 4000
Glen Iris
Victoria 3146
Australia
Tel: 00 61 3 9885 0855
(free catalogue of useful materials)

WABA (World Alliance for Breastfeeding Action)
PO Box 1200
Penang
Malaysia
Tel: 0060 4 6584816

Appendix 3: Breastfeeding initiatives in the UK

The Joint Breastfeeding Initiative

In 1980 and 1985, the Office of Population Censuses and Surveys (OPCS) carried out their second and third investigations into 'Infant Feeding' in the UK (Martin & Monk 1982, Martin & White 1988). Both studies showed a decline in breastfeeding rates from birth to 6 weeks post partum: from 67% at birth to 42% at 6 weeks in 1980 and from 65% at birth to 40% at 6 weeks in 1985. This decline became known as 'the lost 25%'.

It was also clear from the report that the majority of women were stopping earlier than they would have liked because of problems that ought to have been preventable or easily resolved. These findings became the catalyst which generated government support for a 4-year project, the Joint Breastfeeding Initiative (JBI), which was launched at a symposium at the King's Fund Centre in London on 18th October 1988, with representatives from voluntary breastfeeding groups and all health professional organisations from all over the country.

A National Steering Group was set up which was chaired by Barbara Henry, a National Childbirth Trust breastfeeding counsellor. Dora Henschel, a senior health professional, was appointed by the Minister of Health as National Co-ordinator. The Steering Group was made up of representatives from all the health professional organisations whose members were involved in some way with breastfeeding mothers, as well as representatives of the (then) three voluntary breastfeeding support groups. (The representatives were chosen by their own organisations.) The Department of Health also sent observers to attend the Steering Group meetings.

One of the main objectives of the JBI was to encourage District Health Authorities (DHAs) to set up local multidisciplinary breastfeeding working groups, whose composition reflected that of the National Steering Group. To this end the Department of Health published a booklet, 'Supporting and Promoting Breastfeeding: A National Initiative' in which it suggested that the groups might:

- review the local breastfeeding guidelines and revise them as needed
- ensure that local policies were made known to all concerned with the breastfeeding mother and those who gave her support
- enable those policies to be put into action
- provide a means of monitoring those policies
- review the need for education of healthcare staff, other professionals (especially teachers), and the public at large
- collaborate with other bodies to meet local educational needs
- raise public awareness of breastfeeding as the best way of feeding babies.

At the end of the 4-year period of the JBI, a questionnaire was sent to the Chair of each of the 141 local breastfeeding working groups that had been set up, to find out how many of these suggestions they had acted upon. The results showed that the groups had had their greatest impact in the area of public awareness. This was possibly because of the introduction of the national 'Breastfeeding Awareness Week', which has remained an annual event since 1990 and which is funded by the Department of Health.

The groups had also been successful in the development or updating of local breastfeeding guidelines, with four-fifths of DHAs having updated their guidelines on research-based information (RCM 1991).

Reviewing the need for breastfeeding education had been much more difficult. In most DHAs some in-service training had been given, but only ten DHAs had actually introduced training for all midwifery staff, following the introduction of new guidelines. The length of the training varied from 2 to 28 hours.

The importance of in-service training for staff when new guidelines are being implemented cannot be overstated. It is also necessary that attendance at this training be compulsory, and this has implications for service budgets.

The National Breastfeeding Working Group

The main achievement of the JBI in the 4 years of its existence, that of raising the profile of breastfeeding, was acknowledged in the government publication 'The Health of the Nation'

(Secretary of State for Health 1992) which paved the way for the successor to the JBI, the National Breastfeeding Working Group, which held its first meeting in March 1993. Its members, which this time included officers from the Department of Health with a senior officer as chairman, were all appointed by the Department of Health.

With financial support from the Department of Health, the Group maintained the Breastfeeding Awareness Week and supported the existing (JBI) breastfeeding groups with their local efforts in that week. It also relaunched the JBI newsletter in an attempt to keep the local groups in touch.

The (S)JBI continued to flourish in Scotland until October 1995, when it disbanded and the Scottish Breastfeeding Group was formed to carry forward and build on its work. The Health Education Board Scotland (HEBS) took over the support of Breastfeeding Awareness Week in Scotland and a new National Breastfeeding Adviser for Scotland, Jenny Warren, was appointed. As well as providing advice, training resources and support to NHS personnel and lay workers in their efforts to achieve their breastfeeding targets, she also acts as a facilitator to the established Local Joint Breastfeeding Initiatives in Scotland.

In May 1994 the Department of Health funded two fact-finding days as part of an initiative to improve the training of health professionals. The purpose of this exercise was to provide a basis for the production of a new training package called 'Invest in Breast Together', a joint venture between the Royal College of Midwives and the Health Visitors Association. This learning pack was intended to train effective breastfeeding trainers.

In May 1995 the National Breastfeeding Working Group completed, and the Department of Health published, 'Breastfeeding: A Summary of Educational Resources', and 'Breastfeeding: Good Practice, Guidance to the NHS' and in June 1995 the working group was wound up.

The National Network of Breastfeeding Co-ordinators

On 26 May 1995 the Department of Health established the National Network of Breastfeeding Co-ordinators with representatives from each of the eight NHS regions. The voluntary and professional organisations are also represented on the Network. This network, which is currently chaired by the National Infant Feeding Advisers, exists as a mechanism for channelling information on issues of infant feeding nationally and locally.

The Infant Feeding Initiative

In May 1999, as part of the government's new agenda to tackle the health inequalities highlighted in the Acheson Report (1998), the Department of Health set up the Infant Feeding Initiative and this included the appointment of two National Infant Feeding Advisers (Christine Carson, Midwife and Rosemary Thompson, Health Visitor). These posts have been set up for the duration of three years (1999–2002) and will look at ways of improving breastfeeding rates, particularly amongst those women least likely to breastfeed, and thereby reduce the inequalities in breastfeeding.

The UNICEF/WHO Baby-Friendly Initiative UK

This global initiative was developed following a (32-page) Joint Statement of UNICEF and WHO (1989) entitled 'Protecting, Promoting and Supporting Breastfeeding: the special role of maternity services'. The 'Ten Steps to Successful Breastfeeding' contained in this publication and set out here in Appendix 1 formed the basis of the 'Baby-Friendly Hospital Initiative' (BFHI), which was launched, internationally, in June 1991 at the International Pediatric Association Conference in Ankara. In order to become 'Baby Friendly', hospitals have to demonstrate to a team of independent assessors that they fully implement both the Ten Steps and the International Code on the Marketing of Breastmilk Substitutes. (To date more than 14,000 hospitals worldwide have received the UNICEF/WHO 'Baby-Friendly Hospital' award.)

The UNICEF/WHO Baby-Friendly Initiative was launched in the UK in November 1994, with the publication of a 'Mother's Charter: Protecting Breastfeeding Rights'. In 1995 The Royal Bournemouth Hospital became Britain's first Baby-Friendly Hospital, and in the next 5 years over 30 hospitals achieved Baby-Friendly status. In 1998 the Baby-Friendly Initiative was extended into the community and in 2000 Charnwood Surgery, Derby, became the first community healthcare facility to achieve Baby-Friendly accreditation.

The UNICEF UK Baby-Friendly Initiative continues to provide a framework for the implementation of best practice by NHS Trusts and other healthcare facilities. Those which meet the required standard can apply to be assessed and accredited as Baby Friendly. However, information, support and guidance on introducing best practice standards are available to all health facilities and health professionals, regardless of whether they wish to achieve accreditation.

Full details are available from:
UNICEF UK Baby-Friendly Initiative
Africa House
64–78 Kingsway
London WC2B 6NB
Tel: 020 7312 7652
Website: www.babyfriendly.org.uk

References

Acheson D. Independent inquiry into inequalities in health. London: The Stationery Office; 1998.

Martin J, Monk J. Infant feeding 1980. Office of Population Censuses and Surveys. London: HMSO; 1982.

Martin J, White A. Infant feeding 1985. Office of Population Censuses and Surveys. London: HMSO; 1988.

National Breastfeeding Working Group. Breastfeeding: a summary of educational resources. London: Department of Health; 1995.

National Breastfeeding Working Group. Breastfeeding: good practice, guidance to the NHS. London: Department of Health; 1995.

Royal College of Midwives. Successful breastfeeding. 2nd edn. Edinburgh: Churchill Livingstone; 1991.

Secretary of State for Health. The health of the nation. A strategy for health in England. London: HMSO. 1992.

UNICEF/WHO. Mother's charter: protecting breastfeeding rights. London: UNICEF UK Baby-Friendly Initiative; 1994.

World Health Organization. Protecting, promoting and supporting breastfeeding: the special role of maternity services. Geneva: World Health Organization; 1989. Available from HMSO Publications Centre, 51 Nine Elms Lane, London, SW8 5DR.

Appendix 4: Further reading

Alexander J, Levy V, Roch S, series eds. Midwifery Practice series: 'Antenatal care' and 'Postnatal care' (both contain research-based information on breastfeeding). London: Macmillan Education; 1989.

Chalmers I, Enkin M, Keirse NJC, eds. Effective care in pregnancy and childbirth. Oxford: Oxford University Press 1989: chapters 21, 80, 81.

Department of Health and National Breastfeeding Working Group. Breastfeeding: good practice, guidance to the NHS. London: HMSO: 1995 (available from the Department of Health, Room 651C, Skipton House, 80 London Road, London SE1 6LW, UK; tel: 0207 972 2000.)

Greasley V. Breastfeeding. Nursing – the add-on journal of clinical nursing. 3rd series. 1986; 3(2). 63–70.

Inch S. Breastfeeding update In: Alexander J, Levy V, Roch S, eds. Midwifery practice core topics 3. London: Macmillan Education; 2000; 66–82.

Inch S, Fisher C. Breastfeeding: into the 21st century. Nursing Times clinical monograph no. 32. London: EMAP Healthcare; 1999.

La Leche League International. The art of breastfeeding. Australia and London: August Robertson; 1988. The anglicised version of 'The womanly art of breastfeeding'. USA: LLLI; 1981 (available from La Leche League; see Appendix 2).

Minchin M. Breastfeeding matters. Australia: Alma Publications, Allen & Unwin; 1998 (obtainable direct from: PO Box 39, Wendouree, Victoria 3355, Australia; obtainable in the UK from the National Childbirth Trust – see Appendix 2).

Renfrew M, Fisher C, Arms S. Bestfeeding: getting breastfeeding right for you. An illustrated guide. 2nd edn. Berkley, California: Celestial Arts; 2000 (available from Dept B, Airlift Book Company, 26–28 Eden Grove, London N7 8EF, UK).

Breast or bottle? Informed choice leaflets on infant feeding. These and nine other pairs of leaflets (one written for pregnant women, the other for health professionals) are available from: MIDIRS and the NHS Centre for Reviews and Dissemination; tel: freephone 0800 581009.

Videos

Mark-It TV. Breastfeeding – dealing with the problems; 1997 (produced and distributed by Mark-It TV, 7 Quarry Way,

Stapleton, Bristol BS16 1UP, UK; tel: 0117 939 1117. website: www.MarkitTV.com).

Royal College of Midwives. Helping a mother to breastfeed – no finer investment; 1990 (produced and distributed by Healthcare Productions Ltd, Unit 301, Blackfriars Foundry, 156 Blackfriars Road, London SE1 8EN, UK).

Royal College of Midwives. Breastfeeding; coping with the first week; 1996 (produced and distributed by Mark-It TV, 7 Quarry Way, Stapleton, Bristol BS16 1UP, UK; tel: 0117 939 1117).

Appendix 5: Health benefits of breastfeeding

Adapted from the UNICEF UK Baby-Friendly Initiative website.

There has been significant reliable evidence produced over recent years to show that breastfeeding has important advantages for both infant and mother, even in the industrialised countries of the world. Below is a selected list of recently published studies describing differences in health outcome associated with method of infant feeding. The studies have all been adjusted for social and economic variables. All were conducted in an industrialised setting.

Also provided is a list of additional health issues with which breastfeeding has been associated by some researchers. Many of these require further investigation to clarify any protective effect of breastfeeding and are included here for the interest and information of readers.

Artificially fed babies are at greater risk of:

Gastrointestinal infections

Howie PW et al. Protective effect of breast feeding against infection. BMJ 1990; 300(6716): 11–16.

Respiratory infections

Wilson AC et al. Relation of infant diet to childhood health: seven year follow up cohort of children in Dundee infant feeding study. BMJ 1998; 316:21–25.

Wright AL et al. Breast feeding and lower respiratory tract illness in the first year of life. BMJ 1989; 299:946–949.

Necrotising enterocolitis

Lucas A, Cole TJ. Breast milk and neonatal necrotising enterocolitis. Lancet 1990; 336:1519–1522.

Urinary tract infections

Pisacane A, Graziano L, Zona G. Breastfeeding and urinary tract infection. J Pediatr 1992; 120:87–89.

Ear infections

Aniansson G et al. A prospective cohort study on breast feeding and otitis media in Swedish infants. Pediatr Infect Dis J 1994; 13:183–188.

Duncan B et al. Exclusive breast feeding for at least 4 months protects against otitis media. Pediatrics 1993; 5:867–887.

Paradise JL, Elster BA, Tan L. Evidence in infants with cleft palate that breast milk protects against otitis media. Pediatrics 1994; 94:853–860.

Allergic disease (eczema, asthma and wheezing)

Lucas A et al. Early diet of preterm infants and development of allergic or atopic disease: randomised prospective study. BMJ 1990; 300:837–840.

Oddy WH et al. Association between breastfeeding and asthma in 6 year old children: findings of a prospective birth cohort study. BMJ 1999; 319:815 819.

Saarinen UM, Kajosaari M. Breastfeeding as prophylaxis against atopic disease: prospective follow-up study until 17 years old. Lancet 1995; 346:1065 1069.

Wilson AC et al. Relation of infant diet to childhood health: seven year follow up cohort of children in Dundee infant feeding study. BMJ 1998; 316:21–25.

Wright AL et al. Relationship of infant feeding to recurrent wheezing at age 6 years. Arch Pediatr Adolesc Med 1995; 149:758–763.

Insulin-dependent diabetes mellitus

Gerstein HC. Cows' milk exposure and type 1 diabetes mellitus. Diabetes Care 1994; 17:13–19.

Karjalainen J et al. A bovine albumin peptide as a possible trigger of insulin-dependent diabetes mellitus. N Engl J Med 1992; 327:302–307.

Mayer EJ et al. Reduced risk of IDDM among breast-fed children. The Colorado IDDM Registry. Diabetes 1998; 37:1625–1632.

Paronen J et al. Effect of cow's milk exposure and maternal type 1 diabetes on cellular and humoral immunization to dietary insulin in infants at genetic risk for type 1 diabetes. Finnish Trial to Reduce IDDM in the Genetically at Risk Study Group. Diabetes 2000; 49:1657–1665.

Virtanen SM et al. Infant feeding in children <7 years of age with newly diagnosed IDDM. Diabetes Care 1991; 14:415–417.

Breastfed babies may have better:

Neurological development

Anderson JW et al. Breastfeeding and cognitive development: a meta-analysis. Am J Clin Nutr 1999; 70:525–535.

Lucas A et al. Breastmilk and subsequent intelligence quotient in children born preterm. Lancet 1992; 339:261–264.

Morrow-Tlucak M, Haude RH, Ernhart CB. Breastfeeding and cognitive development in the first two years of life. Soc Sci Med 1998; 26:71–82.

Women who breastfed are at lower risk of:

Premenopausal breast cancer

Furberg H et al. Lactation and breast cancer risk. Int J Epidemiol 1999; 28:396–402.

Layde PM et al. The independent associations of parity, age at first full term pregnancy, and duration of breastfeeding with the risk of breast cancer. Cancer and Steroid Hormone Study Group. J Clin Epidemiol 1989; 42:963–973.

Newcomb PA et al. Lactation and a reduced risk of premenopausal breast cancer. N Engl J Med 1994; 330:81–87.

UK National Case–Control Study Group. Breast feeding and risk of breast cancer in young women. BMJ 1993; 307:17–20.

Ovarian cancer

Gwinn ML et al. Pregnancy, breast feeding, and oral contraceptives and the risk of epithelial ovarian cancer. J Clin Epidemiol 1990; 43:559–568.

Rosenblatt KA et al. Lactation and the risk of epithelial ovarian cancer – the WHO Collaborative Study of Neoplasia and Steroid Contraceptives. Int J Epidemiol 1993; 22:499–503.

Hip fractures and reduced bone density

Cumming RG, Klineberg RJ. Breastfeeding and other reproductive factors and the risk of hip fractures in elderly women. Int J Epidemiol 1993; 22:684–691.

Kalkwarf HJ. Hormonal and dietary regulation of changes in bone density during lactation and after weaning in women. J Mammary Gland Biol Neoplasia 1999; 4:319–329.

Kalkwarf HJ, Specker BL. Bone mineral loss during lactation and recovery after weaning. Obstet Gynecol 1995; 86:26–32.

Melton LJ III et al. Influence of breastfeeding and other reproductive factors on bone mass later in life. Osteoporos Int 1993; 3:76–83.

Polatti F et al. Bone mineral changes during and after lactation. Obstet Gynecol 1993; 94:52–56.

Sowers M et al. Changes in bone density with lactation. JAMA 1993; 269:3130–3135.

Sowers M et al. A prospective study of bone density and pregnancy after an extended period of lactation with bone loss. Obstet Gynecol 1995; 85:285–289.

Other studies of health and breastfeeding

Cardiovascular disease in later life

Marmot MG et al. Effect of breast-feeding on plasma cholesterol and weight in young adults. J Epidemiol Community Health 1980; 34:164–167.

Ravelli AC et al. Infant feeding and adult glucose tolerance, lipid profile, blood pressure, and obesity. Arch Dis Child 2000; 82:248–252.

von Kries R et al. Breastfeeding and obesity: cross sectional study. BMJ 1999; 319:147–150.

Wilson AC et al. Relation of infant diet to childhood health: seven year follow up cohort of children in Dundee infant feeding study. BMJ 1998; 316:21–25.

Childhood cancer

Davis MK. Review of the evidence for an association between infant feeding and childhood cancer. Int J Cancer Suppl 1998; 11:29–33.

Mathur GP et al. Breastfeeding and childhood cancer. Indian Pediatr 1993; 30:651–657.

Shu XO et al. Breast-feeding and risk of childhood acute leukemia. J Natl Cancer Inst 1999; 91:1765–1772.

Other potential protective effects of breastfeeding (more research needed)

For the infant:

Multiple sclerosis
Pisacane A et al. Breast feeding and multiple sclerosis. BMJ 1994; 308:1411–1412.

Acute appendicitis

Pisacane A et al. Breast feeding and acute appendicitis. BMJ 1995: 310:836–837.

Tonsillectomy

Pisacane A et al. Breast feeding and tonsillectomy. BMJ 1996; 312:746–747.

For the mother:
Rheumatoid arthritis

Brun JG, Nilssen S, Kvale G. Breast feeding, other reproductive factors and rheumatoid arthritis. A prospective study. Br J Rheumatol 1995; 34(6): 542–546.

Index

A

Abscess, breast, 119
Addresses of voluntary organisations, 135–7
Advice on first feeds, 60–2
Afterpains, 26
Allergic reaction to milk substitutes, 81, 94, 147
Amino acids, 6
Ampullae, 23
Antenatal classes, 94
Antenatal preparation of breast, 96
Antibiotics/antimicrobials for mastitis, 107–8, 109–10
Anticoagulant therapy, 117
Appendicitis, 150
Appetite
 infant's, 39
 mother's, 84
Areola, amount visible, 50, 52
Attachment of baby
 correct, 28–33, 56
 incorrect, 32, 37, 39, 41
 indications of correct, 49–51
 steps to achieving correct, 43–8

B

Baby/infant
 appetite and intake variability, 39
 caesarian section-born, 126
 contact with mother, 55, 60–1, 95
 fluids for, 78–81
 health risks of bottle feeding for, 14–15
 in non-maternity units, 131
 monitoring health and wellbeing, 69–73
 positioning see Positioning
 preterm, 124–5
 sleeping place, 76–9
 stripping of milk by, 27
 sucking see Sucking
 supporting, 45, 46, 48
 twins and triplets, 126–7
 vomiting blood, 115
Baby Friendly Hospital Initiative, 92, 142
Banking, milk, 127–8
Bedding in, 67–9
Benefits of breastfeeding, health, 146–50
Blood
 in milk/colostrum, 115–16
 vomiting of, by baby, 115
Bone density, 148–9
Bottle-feeding
 breastmilk by, 125, 130
 different appearance of, 41–3
 disadvantages of, 14–16
 economics of, 16–18
 milk tokens for, 89
 see also Substitutes, breastmilk
Bowel movements see Stools
Breast
 abscess, 199
 antenatal preparation, 96
 one or both offered, 50, 64
 postnatal care, 98–9
 pregnancy and parturition-related changes, 33
 supporting, 31, 47
 variations in size, 33–4
Breast pump, 100, 127–9
Breastfeed
 influencing decision to, 93–4
 sustaining decision to, 95–6
Breastfeeding
 less common problems, 115–22
 physiology of see Physiology
 prevention of problems, 96–8
 tandem, 119

Breastfeeding (*Contd.*)
  under special circumstances,
    124–31
Breastfeeding initiatives in UK,
    138–42
Breastmilk *see* Milk

C
Caesarian section, 126
Calcium, 9
Calories for mother, additional,
    83–4
Cancer
  breast, 15, 148
  childhood, 149
  ovarian, 148
Carbohydrate, 8–9
Cardiovascular disease, 149
Casein, 5, 6
Central Midwives Board rules, xxi
Childbirth, breast changes during,
    33–4
Cholesterol, 6
Cleanliness, breast, 98
Cleft lip and palate, 118
Colostrum, xix
  blood in, 115–16
  explaining composition to mother,
    62
  expression, 97–8
  storage, 129
  substances contained in, 14
  volume, 24–5
Comparison chart (RCM), 3–4, 5, 8,
    152–153
Complementary feeds, 78–81
Compression, waves/cycles of, 30
Contact dermatitis, 117
Contact of baby with mother, 55,
    60–1, 95
Contraceptive effect of breastfeeding,
    15–16, 66–7
Copper, 9
Cot deaths, 68
Cow's milk, xxi
  allergic reactions, 81
Creams for breast, 98–9
Crying
  incorrect attachment and, 41
  with hunger, 53
Cup-feeding, 130

D
Decision to breastfeed *see*
    Breastfeed
Defaecation *see* Stools
Dehydration, 78
Delivery room, first feed in, 61
Dermatitis, contact, 117
Dextrose supplement, 79
Diabetes, 4–5, 117, 147
Diarrhoea, 25
Diet, breastfeeding mother's, 82–4
Digestive disorders, xix
Donor milk, 125–6
Down syndrome, 119
Drugs and breastfeeding, 117–18
Duration of feeds, xv, 36–7
  unrestricted, 63–4

E
Ear infections, 147
Economic factors in bottle-feeding,
    16–18
Electric pump, 100, 127–9
Engorgement, 103
  milk, 27, 66, 104–8
  prevention, 104–105
  treatment, 105
  vascular, 103–104
Entero-mammary circulation, 13
Epilepsy, 117
Expression
  colostrum, 97–8
  electric pump, 127–9
  hand, 102–3

F
Faeces *see* Stools
Father encouraging breastfeeding,
    95
Fatty acids, 6–8
Feed(s)
  advice and support at first, 60–2
  duration *see* Duration
  frequency *see* Frequency
  mother's position/posture, 53–7
  night time *see* Night

suggestions for first, 53
supplementary, 78–81
unrestricted, 63–6
see also Breastfeed; Breastfeeding
Feedback inhibition of lactation,
27–8, 104
Fertility and breastfeeding, 15–16
First feed *see* Feed(s)
Fluids, additional
for babies, 78–81
for mothers, 82–3
hazards of, 80–1
Free samples of breastmilk
substitutes, 89
Frequency of feeds, 37–9
unrestricted, 64–6

G
Gastrointestinal infections, 17, 146
General health, vital signs of baby's,
73
Growth pattern and weight
measurements, 71

H
Hand, mother's use of left or right,
47
Hand expression, 102–3, 128
Hand pump, 128
Head position, baby's, 43, 45, 47
Health, monitoring baby's, 69–73
Health benefits of breastfeeding,
146–50
Help (to/for mother), 50, 95,
102–3, 128–9
direct ways of giving, 51–7
factors shown not to, 78–84
factors shown to, 60–73
Hepatitis B and C, 121
Herpes simplex infection, 121–2
Hip fractures, 148–9
HIV
breastfeeding and, 120–1
milk banking and, 125–6
Hormones
antidiuretic, 5
lactational, 23–4
Hygiene, personal, 98
Hypoglycaemia, 79–80

I
Immunological factors in breastmilk,
12–13
Infant *see* Baby/infant
Infant Feeding Initiative, 141
Infant Formula and Follow-on
Formula Regulations (1995),
91–2
Infections, 120–2
artificially fed babies and, 146–7
breast pumps as source of, 128
nipple, 116–17
Intake by infant, variability, 39
International voluntary
organisations, 136–7
Iron, 2–3

J
Jaundice, 79
Jaw action, baby's, 32, 50, 52
Joint Breastfeeding Initiative, 138–9,
140

L
Labour, breast changes during, 33–4
Lactation *see* Milk
Lactational amenorrhea method of
contraception, 67
Lactiferous sinuses, 31
Lactose, 8–9
LC-PUFAs in breastmilk substitutes,
7
Let-down reflex, 27–8, 105
Lip, baby's, 45
cleft, 118
Lying down, feeding whilst, 53–6

M
Mammary surgery, 118
Mastitis, 105
antibiotic therapy, 109–10
effective milk removal, 109
infective, 106
non-infective, 106
prevention, 105–7
supportive counselling, 108
treatment, 107–8, 110
Meconium, 72, 73
Methionine, 6

Milk, breast
  banking, 120, 125–6
  blood in, 115–16
  changes in composition, 28, 62
  ejection reflex, 27–8, 120
  engorgement, 66, 104–8
  establishment with electric pump,
    127
  explaining composition to mother,
    28, 62
  night production, 66
  overproduction, 64
  production, 23–4
  release, 28
  removal, 25–7, 28, 109
  storage, 129–30
  substances contained in, 14
  substitutes see Substitutes,
    breastmilk
  volume, 25, 26
Milk tokens for bottle feeding, 89
Minerals, 9
Monitoring baby's health and well-
    being, 69–73
Mortality rate, xix
Mother
  additional calories for, 83–4
  additional fluids for, 82–3
  contact of baby with, 55, 60–1,
    95
  dieting prohititions for, 84
  disadvantages of bottle feeding
    for, 15–16
  helping the see Help
  left or right hand use, 47
  posture, 53–7
  sleeping, 69
Multiple births, 126–7
Multiple sclerosis, 149

N
National Breastfeeding Working
    Group, 139–40
National Network Breastfeeding Co-
    ordinators, 140–1
National voluntary organisations,
    135–6
Neck position baby's, 47
Necrotising enterocolitis, 146

Neurological development, 148
Night feeds, 66–9
  bedding in, 67–9
  mother's sleep, 69
  rooming in, 67
Nipple(s)
  blanching, 116
  infections, 116–17
  inverted, 97, 119–20
  preparation, 97
  shape, 33, 97
  soreness, 37, 96, 98, 99, 116–17
  teat formation, 30, 32
  treatment of sore, 99–102
Nipple confusion, 130
Nipple shields, 99–100, 101–2
Nose, baby's, 45, 46–7
Nutrients, changes in breastmilk of,
    28

O
Oils in breastmilk substitutes, 3
Ointments for breast, 98–9
Otitis media, 15, 16
Ovulation, prolactin levels
    suppressing, 66
Oxytocin release, 23, 25–6, 69,
    104

P
Pain
  after-, 26
  as warning sign, 32
  breast, 50, 98
  milk ejection, 27
Palate, cleft, 118
Parturition, breast changes during,
    33–4
Physiology of breastfeeding, 43, 62,
    65, 96
Pillows, supporting, 56–7
Positioning
  of baby, 28–30, 43
  of mother, 53–7
Postnatal considerations, 98–110
Posture
  midwife's, 57–8
  mother's, 53–7
Pregnancy

breast changes during, 33–4
colostrum expression in, 97–8
Preterm infants, 124–5
Prolactin levels, 23
night feeds and, 66
ovulation suppression and, 66
Protein
human whey, 4, 5, 27
in breastmilk substitutes, 4–6
Psychological components of successful
breastfeeding, 60, 61
Pump
breast, 100, 127–9
hand, 128

R
Reading, further, 114, 133, 144
Reflex
ejection, 27 8, 120
rooting, 28
Repositioning, 100–1
Respiratory infections, 146
Resting and expressing, 100–1
Rheumatoid arthritis, 150
Risks to artificially fed babies, 146–7
Risks to mothers who do not
breastfeed, 148
Rooming in, 67
Rooting reflex, 28, 29
Royal College of Midwives
comparison chart, 3–4, 5, 8,
152–153

S
Scissor grip, discouraging, 48
Scottish Breastfeeding Group, 140
Silicone inserts for pump kits, 129
Sitting up, feeding whilst, 56–7
Sleeping
baby's location, 67–9
by mother, 69
Soreness, nipple *see* Nipple
Soya-based formula, allergic
reactions, 81
Stools, 72–3, 84
blood in, 115
storage of breastmilk, 129–30
Substitutes, breastmilk
bioavailability, 10

biological differences, 10
carbohydrate in, 8–9
cholesterol in, 6
compared with breast milk, 3–4
composition, 2–3
controlling intake, 12
errors during manufacture,
10–11
errors during preparation, 11–12
fatty acids in, 6–8
free amino acids in, 6
free samples, 89
immunological factors, 12–13
limitations of, 1–2
minerals in, 9
nutritional summary, 12
oils in, 3
promotion, 90–2
protein in, 4 6
trace elements in, 9
see also Bottle-feeding
Sucking by infant, 28–33
cycle, 30
explaining to mother, 28, 32
in bottle-feeding versus
breastfeeding, 41–3
limiting time of, 63, 99
Supplementary feeds, 78–81
Support (encouragement) with
breastfeeding 95–6
at first feed, 60–2
Support (physical)
of baby, 48
of breast, 47
of mother, 50–1
Surgery, mammary, 118

T
Tandem feeding, 119
Taurine, 2, 7
Ten steps to successful breastfeeding,
62, 92, 134, 141–2
Thrush infection of nipple,
116–17
Tongue, baby's, 31–2, 52
Tonsillectomy, 150
Trace elements, 9
Triplets, 127
Twins, 126–7

U

UNICEF/WHO Baby-Friendly
    Initiative UK, 92, 141–2
Urinary tract infections, 146

V

Vascular engorgement, 103
Videos on breastfeeding, 144–5
Voluntary organisations, national and
    international, 135–7
Vomiting of blood by baby, 115

W

Weighing, test, 81–2

Weight, baby's
    failure to gain, 64
    gain, 65, 70–1
    variations, 71–2
Weight, mother's, 83–4
Well-being, monitoring baby's,
    69–73
White nipple, 116
WHO Code for the Marketing of
    Breastmilk Substitutes,
    90–1

Z

Zinc, 9